New immunomodulating agents
and biological response modifiers

Human cancer immunology

Volume 3

Elsevier Biomedical Press
Amsterdam · New York · Oxford

New immunomodulating agents and biological response modifiers

edited by

B. Serrou

Laboratoire d'Immunopharmacologie des Tumeurs,
INSERM U-236, ERA-CNRS No. 844,
Centre Paul Lamarque,
BP 5054, 34033 Montpellier, France

and

C. Rosenfeld

ICIG, Hôpital Paul Brousse,
14-16 Ave. Paul Vaillant Couturier,
94800 Villejuif, France

Guest editors

J. Wybran   *and*   G. Meyer

Hôpital Erasme,   *Institut Paoli-Calmettes, CRAM 232,*
Service d'Immunohematologie 0808,   *Bld de Ste Marguerite, 13273 Marseille,*
Route de Leenick, 1070 Bruxelles, Belgium   *France*

1982
Elsevier Biomedical Press
Amsterdam · New York · Oxford

ISBN series: 0 444 80236 3
ISBN volume 3: 0 444 80401 3

Published by:

Elsevier Biomedical Press B.V.
P.O. Box 211
1000 AZ Amsterdam,
The Netherlands

Sole distributors for the U.S.A. and Canada:

Elsevier Science Publishing Company Inc.,
52 Vanderbilt Avenue,
New York, NY 10017,
U.S.A.

Library of Congress Cataloging in Publication Data
Main entry under title:

New immunomodulating agents and biological response
    modifiers.

    (Human cancer immunology ; v. 3)
    "Contains the lectures presented on September 29, 1980
at the Erasme Hospital, University of Brussels by the
Tumor Immunology Project Group (TIPG)"--Foreword.
    Bibliography: p.
    Includes index.
    1. Immunotherapy--Congresses. 2. Cancer--Chemotherapy
--Congresses. 3. Immune response--Regulation--Congresses.
I. Serrou, Bernard. II. Rosenfeld, C. (Claude)
III. Series. [DNLM: 1. Neoplasms--Drug therapy.
2. Neoplasms--Immunology. 3. Adjuvants, Immunologic--
Therapeutic use. 4. Antineoplastic agents--Therapeutic
use. WI HU444WF v.3 / QZ 267 N5325]
RC271.I45N48   616.99'4061   82-2433
ISBN 0-444-80401-3   AACR2

Printed in the Netherlands

Foreword

This book, as the third in the series on 'Human Cancer Immunology', contains the lectures presented on September 29 1980 at the Erasme Hospital, University of Brussels by the Tumor Immunology Project Group (TIPG). The aim of the meeting was the review of some drugs with immunomodulatory properties by major contributors in the field. It was also considered that this meeting would help in the development of the further strategy of the TIPG.

Indeed, one of the goals of the TIPG is the screening of various drugs for their possible properties as modifiers of the biological response and for their immunological properties. The Brussels meeting was thus organized in such a way that the presentation of the various drugs was followed by a discussion of all the members, in order to select a drug to be tested by the TIPG.

After one drug had been chosen, the TIPG members structured a phase I – phase II trial to define, in cancer patients, the optimal dosage of the drug that is able to modulate the immune response of these patients. This work is currently in progress. Obviously this approach is based on the hypothesis that immunomodulation by synthetic drugs alone or in combination with other forms of cancer treatment should lead to an improvement in the treatment of cancer patients. In these recent years, well-controlled clinical trials, with conditions such as acute myeloblastic leukemia, lung cancer, lymphomas, metastatic breast cancer, metastatic ovary cancer and bladder carcinoma, have shown that non-specific immunomodulation increases the length of remissions and improves the survival in the patients. Consequently, since the new techniques allow a better immunological monitoring and the pharmacological industry is continually synthetizing new drugs, the members of the TIPG have the deep conviction that their trials will provide a scientific basis for immunomodulation in cancer treatment.

J. Wybran
President, Tumor Immunology Project Group

B. Serrou
Secretary, Tumor Immunology Project Group

Contributors

M. AL-HASHIMI – Institute for Cancer Research, University of Vienna, Borschke-gasse 8a, A-1090 Vienna, Austria

P. BARDOS – Laboratoire d'Immunologie, Faculté de Médecine, B.P. 3323, 37032 Tours Cédex, France

M. BRULEY–ROSSET – ICIG, INSERM U. 50, Hôpital Paul-Brousse, 14 Avenue Paul Vaillant Couturier, Villejuif, France

J.P. BURET – Laboratoires Cassenne et Centre de Recherche Roussel-UCLAF, Paris, France

B. COLLET – Centre Régional de Lutte contre le Cancer, Rennes, France

M. COLOT – Institute for Cancer Research, University of Vienna, Borschkegasse 8a, A-1090 Vienna, Austria

D. CUPISSOL – Laboratoire d'Immunopharmacologie des Tumeurs, INSERM U-236, ERA-CNRS No. 844, Centre Paul Lamarque, BP 5054, 34 033 Montpellier Cédex, France

C. DAVID – Laboratoire Vétérinaire Départemental, Rennes, France

L. DAZORD – Laboratoire Vétérinaire Départemental, Rennes, France

C. DITTRICH – Clinic for Chemotherapy, Department for Oncology, University of Vienna, Borschkegasse 8a, A-1090 Vienna, Austria

L. DUSSOURD'D'HINTERLAND – Centre d'Immunologie et de Biologie P. Fabre, 17 Av. Jean Moulin, 81 106 Castres, France

C. ESTEVE – Laboratoire d'Immunopharmacologie des Tumeurs, INSERM U-236, ERA-CNRS No. 844, Centre Paul Lamarque, B.P. 5054, 34 033 Montpellier Cédex, France

I. FLORENTIN – ICIG, INSERM U. 50, Hôpital Paul-Brousse, 14 Avenue Paul
Vaillant Couturier, Villejuif, France

A. FRITSCH – I. Department of Surgery, University of Vienna, Borschkegasse 8a,
A-1090 Vienna, Austria

C. GIRON – Service des Maladies du Sang, Hôpital de Hautepierre, 67098
Strasbourg, France

A. GOUTNER – ICIG, INSERM U. 50, Hôpital Paul-Brousse, 14 Avenue Paul
Vaillant Couturier, Villejuif, France

G.R. HEMSWORTH – Pfizer Central Research, Groton, Connecticut 06340, U.S.A.

W.W. HOFFMAN – Pfizer Central Research, Groton, Connecticut 06340, U.S.A.

T. HOSHINO –II Med. Clinic, Department of Medicine, Medical Faculty, Kyoto
University, Japan

R. JAKESZ – Department of Surgery, University of Vienna, Borschkegasse 8a,
A-1090 Vienna, Austria

K.E. JENSEN – Pfizer Central Research, Groton, Connecticut 06340, U.S.A.

E.M. KOKOSCHKA – Department of Dermatology, University of Vienna, Borschkegasse 8a, A-1090 Vienna, Austria

A.R. KRASKA – Pfizer Central Research, Groton, Connecticut 06340, U.S.A.

J.M. LANG – Service des Maladies du Sang, Hôpital de Hautepierre, 67098
Strasbourg, France

Y. LEBRANCHU – Laboratoire d'Immunologie, Faculté de Médecine, B.P. 3223,
37032 Tours Cédex, France

Y. LE GARREC – Institut Pasteur, Paris, France

T. LUGER – II. Department of Dermatology, University of Vienna, Borschkegasse
8a, A-1090 Vienna, Austria

C. MARCHIANI – Laboratoires Cassenne et Centre de Recherche Roussel-UCLAF,
Paris, France

A. MARTIN – Centre Régional de Lutte contre le Cancer, Rennes, France

M. MICKSCHE – Institute for Cancer Research, University of Vienna, Borschkegasse 8a, A-1090 Vienna, Austria

K. MOSER – Clinic for Chemotherapy, Department for Oncology, University of Vienna, Borschkegasse 8a, A-1090 Vienna, Austria

P.G. MUNDER – Max-Planck-Institut für Immunbiologie, Freiburg i.Br., F.R.G.

J.F. NIBLACK – Pfizer Central Research, Groton, Connecticut 96340, U.S.A.

F. NASRAT – ICIG, INSERM U.50, Hôpital Paul-Brousse, 14 Avenue Paul Vaillant Couturier, Villejuif, France

G. NORMIER – Centre d'Immunologie et de Biologie P. Fabre, 17 Av. Jean Moulin, 81 106 Castres, France

F. OBERLING – Service des Maladies du Sang, Hôpital de Hautepierre, 67098 Strasbourg, France

I.G. OTTERNESS – Pfizer Central Research, Groton, Connecticut 96340, U.S.A.

A.M. PINELE – Centre d'Immunologie et de Biologie P. Fabre, 17 Av. Jean Moulin, 81 106 Castres, France

H. RAINER – Clinic for Chemotherapy, Department for Oncology, University of Vienna, Borschkegasse 8a, A-1090 Vienna, Austria

G. RENOUX – Laboratoire d'Immunologie, Faculté de Médecine, B.P. 3223, 37032 Tours Cédex, France

M. RENOUX – Laboratoire d'Immunologie, Faculté de Médecine, B.P. 3223, 37032 Tours Cédex, France

A. REY – Laboratoire d'Immunopharmacologie des Tumeurs, INSERM U 236, ERA-CNRS No. 844, Centre Paul Lamarque, B.P. 5054, 34 033 Montpellier Cédex, France

C. ROSENFELD – Département de Cultures et Production de Cellules Humaines, INSERM U 50, ICIG, Hôpital Paul Brousse, 14-16, Av. P. Vaillant Couturier, 94 800 Villejuif, France

H.D. SCHLUMBERGER – Institute of Immunology and Oncology, Bayer AG, 5600 Wuppertal-1, F.R.G.

B. SERROU – Laboratoire d'Immunopharmacologie des Tumeurs, INSERM U 236, ERA-CNRS No. 844, Centre Paul Lamarque, B.P. 5054, 34 033 Montpellier Cédex, France

N. SIMON-LAVOINE – Laboratoire Servier, 22 rue Garnier, 92200 Neuilly, France

C. THIERRY – Laboratoire d'Immunopharmacologie des Tumeurs, INSERM U 236, ERA-CNRS No. 844, Centre Paul Lamarque, B.P. 5054, 34 033 Montpellier Cédex, France

L. TOUJAS – Centre Régional de Lutte contre le Cancer, F. 35 000, Rennes, France

A. UCHIDA – Institute for Cancer Research, University of Vienna, Borschkegasse 8a, A-1090 Vienna, Austria

J.S. WOLFF III – Pfizer Central Research, Groton, Connecticut 96340, U.S.A.

J. WYBRAN – Department of Immunology, Erasmus Hospital, Free University of Brussels, 808, Route de Lennick, B-1070 Brussels, Belgium

S. YAMAGATA – Institute for Cancer Research, University of Vienna, Borschkegasse 8a, A-1090 Vienna, Austria

R. ZALISZ – Laboratoires Cassenne et Centre de Recherche Roussell-UCLAF, Paris, France.

Contents

CHAPTER 1

Modifications of the biologic response against tumours by *Brucella abortus*

L. Dazord[a], A. Martin[a], B. Collet[a], Y. le Garrec[b], C. David[c], and L. Toujas[a]

[a]*Centre Régional de Lutte Contre le Cancer, Rennes,* [b] *Institut Pasteur, Paris and* [c]*Laboratoire Vétérinaire Départemental, Rennes (France)*

1.1. INTRODUCTION

Brucella abortus, the agent of infectious abortion in cattle, was discovered by Bang in 1896. *B. abortus* is also pathogenic for man. It generally causes less severe infections than those from *B. melitensis*. Infections by *B. abortus* were found to be either chronic or latent through systematic surveys of populations exposed to animal contamination [1].

Brucella strains of attenuated virulence have been prepared for vaccination. The strain B19S proposed by Cotton et al. [2] in 1932 is still widely used for cattle vaccination. However, the strain 19BA which is derived from the B19S strain has been employed for human vaccination [3].

Experimental infection with the 19BA or B19 strains was found to protect mice against the development of various transplantable tumours [4–10]. This prompted us to propose the strain 19BA as an immunotherapeutic agent for cancer patients. It would be, like *Mycobacterium bovis* strain BCG, one of the rare organisms used in the living state for the treatment of human tumours. It is also remarkable that *Mycobacterium* and *Brucella* share common biological properties such as intracellular growth and a tendency to cause chronic infection usually accompanied by granulomata and delayed-type hypersensitivity reactions.

Inactivated *B. abortus* organisms can also delay the growth of experimental tumours [5,11–20]. The mechanisms of this effect has been extensively studied [21–27]. However, *B. abortus* is a Gram negative organism, bearing endotoxins and provoking strong allergic reactions. As judged from experimental data [27], the quantities of dead organisms active on tumours are 100 to 1000 times greater than when using live Brucellae. For these reasons it is thought that the use of inactivated *B. abortus* organisms in man will require a preliminary step of chemical treatment of the bacterium to reduce its toxicity and antigenicity.

Except for the work of Hirnle [4] in 1960, most of the studies on the antitumour activity of *B. abortus* have been reported since 1970. A few major points have been established from the research conducted in the past 10 years and these include the experimental evidence for the antitumour activity of live *B. abortus*; use of the live vaccine 19BA in human immunotherapy; experimental evidence for the antitumour activity of dead *B. abortus* with elaboration on the mechanisms of action; and chemical treatment of the organisms.

1.2. EXPERIMENTAL EVIDENCE FOR THE ANTITUMOUR ACTIVITY OF LIVE *B. abortus* ORGANISMS

Table 1.I summarizes the main work on the antitumour activity of *B. abortus*. Live organisms were studied by different teams using different experimental systems. Pathogenic organisms as well as attenuated strains were found active against tumours.

Table 1.I.

Main experimental works on the antitumour activity of living and inactivated *B. abortus* organisms

Brucella strains	Experimental model (tumours/mice)	Ref.
	(a) Live organisms	
Pathogenic	Sarcoma 108/A,C_{57} R III	4
B19	Erhlich ascite/Swiss	5
19BA	RLV induced/Balb c	
	L1210/DBA$_2$	6
19BA	S 180, melanoma / Swiss, Balb c	7
19BA	Myeloïd leuk. / C57 Bl	8
B19	EL4 lymphoma / B$_6$ D$_2$	9
B19 S/R, 19BA	EL4 lymphoma, Lewis Cα/B6 D2	10
	(b) Inactivated organisms	
B19	Ehrlich / Swiss	5
B19	L 1210 / B6 D2	11
B19	MCA induced / various strains	12
	Spont. leuk / AKR	
Bru-pel	S 180 / Swiss	13
Bru-pel	L1210 / CD$_2$	14
Bru-pel	LSTRA Sa /CD$_2$	15
	M 109 Ca	
Bru-pel	MBL2 Leuk /CD$_2$	16
	M 109 Ca	
Bru-pel	Osteosarcoma / C_{57} Bl	17
Bru-pel	Mamm Ca / C_3H	18
B19S/R	Lewis Ca, Bl6 Mel. /B$_6$ D$_2$	19
	Mamm. Ca., L1210, EL$_4$, MBL$_2$	
B19–NaOH	EL$_4$ lymph. Lewis Ca / B$_6$ D$_2$	20

Early work done in the laboratory utilized strain B19 cultured in smooth phase (B19S). The bacterium was provided by Institut Mérieux (Aborsec Vaccine) and was cultured on soy agar medium. The cultures containing less than 1% rough forms, were collected, washed and kept at −80°C [9]. The organisms were studied in C57 B16/DBA2 (B6 D2) F_1 mice which were challenged with EL 4 lymphoma.

A correlation was found between the intensity of the *Brucella* infection and the resistance against the tumour. B6 D2 mice were infected by iv administration of either 5×10^2 or 5×10^6 viable organisms. The kinetics of the infection were determined by counting the number of organisms in the spleen. The infection with 5×10^6 organisms reached a peak in the first week. Infection with 5×10^2 organisms was peaking on the third week and the number of organisms was lower than after injection of 5×10^6 organisms. In parallel, groups of mice infected with 5×10^2 and 5×10^6 brucellae were challenged with EL4 lymphoma. As shown in Table II there was good correlation between the number of organisms in the spleen and the prolongation of survival after tumour graft.

Table 1.II.

Relationship between intensity of the injection of *B. abortus* B19S and resistance against lymphoma graft

Day 0 injection		Weeks after *B. abortus* injection					
		1	2	3	4	5	6
$5 \times 10^{6^a}$	Bacteria in the spleen [b]	7	6.8	5.7	5.2	3.7	1
	Survival of EL$_4$ grafted [c]	33.0[d]	32.4[d]	27.4	26.6	26.3	25.5
$5 \times 10^{2^b}$	Bacteria in the spleen [b]	4.4	6.0	6.6	5.8	5.0	1
	Survival of EL$_4$ grafted [c]	26.6	26.0	28.6[d]	28.6[d]	27.2[d]	26.2

[a] B19S organisms injected iv.
[b] Number of bacteria per spleen expressed by log 10.
[c] 10^3 EL$_4$ cells grafted ip at the times after *Brucella* injection indicated. Survival time of controls : 25.6 days.
[d] Significantly different from the control group.

Factors affecting the degree of infection were then studied. The role of the strain of bacterium used was investigated by comparing B19R, B19R and 19BA strains. The strain B19R is a rough mutant of B19S selected by culture in fluid medium. The strain 19BA used for human vaccination was kindly provided by the Gameleya Institute (Moscow). Strains B19R and 19BA in S phase were cultured and kept as described for B19S. The kinetics of in vivo growth of the three strains were found to

4

be quite parallel when the organisms were injected intravenously [10]. But when they were inoculated by other routes differences appeared between them. As can be seen in Table 1.III the penetration of the rough organisms was inhibited when using subcutaneous or intradermal routes.

Table 1.III.

Number of organisms in the spleen and liver 7 days after injection of 5×10^6 organisms of various strains of *B. abortus* by various routes

Route of inoculation	B19S		19BA		B19R	
	Spleen	Liver	Spleen	Liver	Spleen	Liver
iv	6.0	5.2	6.9	6.3	6.1	5.4
ip	7.0	5.4	6.9	4.6	5.5	3.2
sc	6.3	4.6	3.7	2.6	2.3	1
id	3.5	2.5	2.2	1	1.4	2.6

The spread of the infection also depended on the local inflammatory reaction. Freund's incomplete adjuvant added to 19BA organisms, then injected subcutaneously increased the number of bacteria present in the spleen. In addition, immunosuppressive drugs, hydrocortisone and cyclophosphamide, resulted in an enhanced proliferation of the organisms (Table 1.IV).

Table 1.IV.

Factors influencing the diffusion of the infection by 5×10^7 19BA organisms injected subcutaneously

ip Injection on Day –2	sc Injection on Day 0	Number of organisms on Day 8	
		Spleen	Liver
None	19BA	2.7	2.6
None	19BA + FIA	4.3	2.6
Hydrocortisone (125 mg/kg^{-1})	19BA	4.4	3.3
Cyclophosphamide (300 mg / kg^{-1})	19BA	5.0	2.9

The effect of live *B. abortus* on EL4 lymphoma was compared with that of BCG, *C. parvum* and killed *B. abortus*. No substantial difference was found between the various organisms. However, when tested on Lewis tumour *B. abortus* was shown to be more effective than BCG [10]. The infection by *B. abortus* was also found to improve the antitumour activity of cyclophosphamide on Lewis tumour.

1.3. TREATMENT OF CANCER PATIENTS WITH VACCINE 19BA

A preliminary clinical trial was undertaken in patients with acute myeloid leukemia or lung cancer. First the negativity of the immune responses against brucellosis was checked by the Wright sero-agglutination test, complement fixation and Melitin skin test. The first patients received the organisms by scarification and the following patients by subcutaneous injection. The doses injected were increased progressively up to 10^{10} organisms. This dose was applied to 18 patients (Table 1.V). In general it was well tolerated, provoked a local swelling of 3 – 5 cm; no adenophathy. The temperature increase did not exceed 38°C the day after brucella injection. Anti-brucella antibodies appeared in most of the patients' sera 7 or 14 days after the bacterial inoculation. Most of the patients underwent an immunosuppressive treatment (radio- or chemotherapy) before *B. abortus* treatment. Only seven of them, treated surgically for a lung carcinoma, did not receive any complementary suppressive treatment. In six of these seven patients *B. abortus* provoked an increase of the number of blood mononuclear cells of 53, 85, 105, 138, 164, 280%. The spleen volume also seemed to increase. It was augmented in five of six patients by 13, 15, 24, 34, 55%. The PHA response, the number of E rosettes and the skin tests did not seem affected by the treatment.

Table 1.V.

Main results of a preliminary trial of live *B. abortus* organisms in cancer patients

No. of patients	No. of bacteria injected s.c.		Local oedema[a]	Fever[b]	Mononuclear cell increase	Spleen hypertrophy	Wright sero-diagnostic
1	$2.5 \ 10^7$		0/1	0/1	0/1	–	0/1
1	$2.5 \ 10^8$		0/1	0/1	0/1	–	0/1
2	10^9		1/2	1/2	1/2	–	1/2
18	10^{10}	Previous chemo- or radiotherapy (11)	8/11	5/11	–	–	6/11
		No chemo- or radiotherapy (7)	7/7	6/7	6/7	5/6	7/7

[a] Oedema of more than 3 cm at the site of injection.
[b] More than 37°C.

1.4. ANTITUMOUR ACTIVITY AND MECHANISMS OF ACTION OF KILLED *B. abortus* ORGANISMS

Table 1.I has shown that *Brucella* preparations derived from strain B19 or preparation Bru-pel derived from the strain 456 were efficient against tumours in various experimental situations.

The organisms were found active when injected before or after tumour graft. Favourable results were obtained when the treatment was applied during the period of induction of virally or chemically induced tumours [12]. The treatment was combined successfully with chemotherapy [15,18].

Some work was carried out to investigate the mechanism of the antitumour effect of heat-killed *B. abortus* organisms. Correlations were sought between the activity on tumours and other biological properties of the bacteria such as: immunostimulant activity, haemotological modifications provoked by iv injections, toxicity of the organisms, and the ability to form granulomas and to activate macrophages.

1.4.1. Immunostimulant properties and antitimour activity

The effect of the iv injection of *B. abortus* B19S was studied on the following responses: (a) the response against sheep red blood cell (SRBC) antigens as measured by the number of spleen plaque forming cells (PFC); (b) the delayed type hypersensitivity (DTH) reaction against SRBC; and (c) the ability of spleen cells to respond in a mixed lymphocyte culture (MLC). The admixture of B19S with SRBC injected intravenously did not increase the number of PFC measured 4 days later in the spleen. In contrast, in animals pre-treated with an anti-B19S antiserum the number of PFC was increased (Table 1.VI). Since it is possible that the administration of antiserum diminished the active production of anti-B19S

Table 1.VI.

Modulation of the antibody response against SRBC by *B. abortus* in various experimental conditions

Expt	Injection on Day −1 (ip)	Injection on Day 0[a] (iv)	Number of PFC on Day 4[b]	
			per spleen	per 10^6 cells
1	Normal serum	SRBC	53 150 ± 4865	352 ± 85
	Normal serum	B19S + SRBC	55 550 ± 2600	315 ± 37
	Anti-B19S antiserum[b]	B19S + SRBC	164 300 ± 11 350	1 136 ± 85
2	None	SRBC	67 500 ± 9250	359 ± 102
	None	B19S + SRBC	73 950 ± 8000	289 ± 75
	None	B19S-anti B19S complex + SRBC	201 250 ± 18 625	719 ± 303
	None	B19R + SRBC	227 500 ± 24 250	823 ± 201

[a] : iv injection of 2.5×10^8 SRBC and 500 μg of *Brucella* preparation.
[b] : 0.1 ml of anti-B19S serum prepared in isologous mice as described in Ref 21.

agglutinins it was suggested that the reduction in the expression of the surface antigens of *B. abortus* resulted in an enhancement of its immunostimulatory activity [21]. This hypothesis was confirmed by using two nonagglutinogenic preparations of *B. abortus;* the B19S – anti-B19S complex and the rough mutant B19R [23]. As shown in Table 1.VI such preparations had immunostimulant properties.

Opposite effects of B19S and B19R on T-dependent immune reactions were also found [24]. The iv injection of B19S strongly depressed DTH to SRBC while B19R did not affect it. Furthermore, B19S depressed MLC in circumstances in which B19R increased it or did not alter it.

The two *Brucella* preparations S and R were studied comparatively on six different tumours (three ascitic, three solid) using six different experimental protocols for treatment [19]. The organisms were either injected locally at the site of tumour implantation or were given by systemic route, 10 days or 5 days before tumour graft or 1 day after. Injection of the bacteria before the graft of solid tumours accelerated tumour growth. Other protocols did not influence significantly the survival of the animals. Almost all the local treatments and those performed after tumour graft prolonged the survival time. B19S gave more favourable results than B19R on the solid tumours and vice versa for the ascitic tumours. But in all cases the two bacteria preparations provoked the same kind of effect. They never acted in opposite ways in a given experimental condition. Table 1.VII shows simplified results concerning only the systemic injection of B19S and B19R. It is

Table 1.VII.

Effect of the iv injection of 500 g of B19S or B19R on immune responses and tumour growth

	PFC[a]	MLC[b]	DTH[b]	Day –5 before graft		Day 1 after graft	
				solid	ascitic	solid	ascitic
S	0	–	–	–	+	+	+
R	+	Ob	O	–	+	+	+

0: no difference   –: diminution   +: augmented response as compared to control.
[a] see ref. 23.   [b] see ref. 24.   [c] see ref 19.

clear that despite opposite effects on T-dependent immune responses the two bacterial preparations exerted parallel effects on tumours. In Figure 1.1, the DTH response 1 – 20 days after iv inoculation of B19S and B19R and the response to the graft of 10^6 EL$_4$ cells by the intravenous route were compared. There was obviously no correlation between the modifications of the T-dependent response against SRBC and the enhancement of the response against the tumour graft. The preparation B19S which depressed DTH, strongly increased the resistance against the lymphoma. The depression of DTH by B19S was maximal at a time when the antitumour response was best enhanced.

8

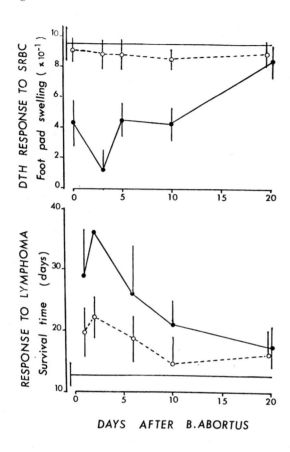

Fig. 1.1. Variations of the DTH response to SRBC and of the survival after lymphoma graft at various times after iv injection of 500 μg of *B. abortus* B19S (●—●) or B19R (○—○). Controls are represented by horizontal bars. The sensitization to SRBC antigens was achieved by iv injection of 10^6 cells and DTH was revealed by a foot pad injection of 10^8 cells. The lymphoma was grafted by iv inoculation of 10^6 cells.

1.4.2 Antitumour activity and haematological modifications following B. abortus injection.

The iv injection of 500 μg *B. abortus*, B19S into $B_6 D_2$ mice provoked important modifications of haematopoiesis. First the number of stem cells diminished in the bone marrow and increased in the spleen, suggesting a migration from one organ to the other. Then the spleen was enriched in blast cells of several types (erythroblasts, megacaryocytes, PMN precursors) and reached its maximal hypertrophy on Day 10. The number of colony forming units (CFU) in bone marrow remained low up to the 20th day but increased on the 40th [22]. This rebound phenomenon of the 40th day was associated with an enhanced resistance against the graft of L 1210 leukemia [11] or of E♂G2 leukemia, as shown in Fig. 1.2.

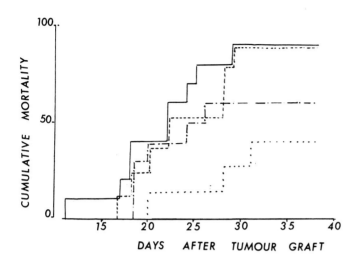

Fig. 1.2. Survival of mice grafted ip with 10^4 E♂ G_2 cells at various times after iv injection of 500 μg of *B. abortus* B19S. Controls, no B19S (–), B19S 10 days before leukemic graft (– – –) 20 days before (–.–) 40 days before (...).

However B19R did not provoke important changes of the spleen weight. Thus, the antitumour effects detected shortly after *Brucella* injection seem to be independent of the effects on haematopoiesis. Later effects could result from the proliferation of bone marrow cells.

1.4.3. Antitumour activity and ability of B. abortus to induce granulomatous reactions and activate macrophages.

The sc injection of B19S and B19R organisms into the foot pad of mice provoked granulomatous reactions which were found histologically to involve mainly histiocytes. It is remarkable that both kinds of bacteria had a comparable aptitude to provoke a granulomatous reaction in the subcutaneous tissue [27] in spite of different capacities to induce spleen hypertrophy.

Both B19S and B19R have been found to activate macrophages of the peritoneal cavity [25]. The process of activation seemed to involve the participation of newly generated macrophages [26]. As shown in Table 1.VIII a good correlation was found between the resistance against an intraperitoneal graft of EL_4 lymphoma and the cytotoxic activity of peritoneal macrophages. Both phenomena peaked 3 or 4 days after *B. abortus* and decreased slowly thereafter. Furthermore, the administration of silica, which is toxic for macrophages, was found to inhibit the antitumour activity of *Brucella* (in preparation).

Table 1.VIII.

Induction of an increased resistance against EL$_4$ lymphoma by ip injection of 500 μg of *B. abortus* B19R. Comparison between in vivo resistance to the ip lymphoma graft and in vitro cytotoxic activity of peritoneal macrophages

	Days after ip injection of 500 μg of B19R								
	Control	0	1	2	3	5	10	14	20
Survival after graft [a]	13.0 ±1.9	15.3 ±2.0	17.1 ±1.6	20.2 ±2.6	21.3 ±3.1	17.6 ±2.9	17.5 ±2.8	16.3 ±2.1	15.3 ±2.2
Cytotoxicity (isotope release) [b]	3047 ±492	–	2549 ±219	3399 ±264	4236 ±85	5368 ±14	3589 ±357	3469 ±238	3243 ±562

[a] 10^6 EL$_4$ cells grafted ip in mice pretreated at various times before with 500 μg of B19R.
[b] Peritoneal macrophages sampled at various times after ip injection of B19R and cultured in the presence of [^{3}H]thymidine–labeled EL$_4$ cells. The cytotoxic activity was assessed by the measurement of the radioactivity released.

1.5. CHEMICAL TREATMENTS OF *B. abortus* ORGANISMS

1.5.1. Extraction by ether

The treatment of *B. abortus* strain 19 by the method of Badakhsh, Foster and Ribi using a mixture of ether and water allowed the extraction of substance with toxic properties [28]. Youngner et al. showed that the substance extracted by ether from *B. abortus* strain 456 had interferon-inducing properties comparable to those of the endotoxin of Gram negative organisms [29]. The bacterial residue, called Bru-pel, lost its ability to induce an endotoxin-like interferon but did exhibit antitumour properties [13]. Thus, a treatment known to extract toxic substances did not alter the effects of *B. abortus* on tumours.

1.5.2. Mild alkaline treatment

Alkaline treatment was first used by Raistrich and Topley [30] to detoxify bacterial endotoxins. We observed that the treatment of *B. abortus* organisms by 0.01 M or 0.02 M NaOH for 24 h at room temperature was optimal to delay the growth of Lewis carcinoma in mice [20]. NaOH–treated bacteria were injected in adrenalectomized mice and the LD 50 was found to increase by 50 – 100 times when compared with untreated organisms. Comparison of NaOH-treated or untreated B19S and B19R on the growth of Lewis tumour and EL$_4$ lymphoma in mice did not attribute important differences to the NaOH treatment. Thus again a diminution of the toxicity of *B. abortus* did not affect its antitumour activity.

1.5.3 Other physico-chemical treatments

B. abortus organisms have been systematically attacked by various chemical reagents [27]. Some of these reagents, such as HCl, ethanol and chloroform, were found to reduce the antitumour activity of *B. abortus*. Other treatments, such as heating at 100°C, ether, which confirmed the experiments on Bru-pel, NaOH 0.01 M, pronase digestion or treatment by hypertonic NaCl did not seem to affect this property. The sequential addition of chemical treatments was found to be possible. As shown in Table 1.IX the addition of ether and NaOH which both lower the toxicity of the bacteria, did not alter the antitumour activity.

Table 1.IX.

Protective effect of *B. abortus* B19R after various treatments

Treatments of B19R organisms	Proportion of survivors	Survival time
No bacteria (controls)	0/30	12.1 ± 0.9
Heating at 65°C	2/8	31.5 ± 8.3
Ether (3 extractions)	2/8	25.1 ± 5.9
NaOH 0.01 M 24 h	5/8	29.3 ± 0.6
Ether + NaOH	5/8	28.6 ± 6.1

500 μg of each *B. abortus* preparation was injected ip 3 days before ip graft of 10^6 EL$_4$ cells.

1.6. DISCUSSION

Live, as well as killed, *Brucella* organisms have been found to be active against tumours in certain experimental models. To be effective in humans very high doses of inactivated *Brucella* would have to be injected in cases of cancer. However, the inherent toxicity of these gram negative bacteria and the strong secondary reactions they can elicit due to their high antigenicity prevent their use as such.

Live *Brucella* have been reported to exert an antitumour activity at low doses where the toxic effect is minimal. Our experimental studies have established the following points. A strong correlation seems to exist between the degree of bacterial infection and the antitumour effect. The iv route induces the strongest infection. The effect of the cutaneous barrier is more marked with B19R than B19S.

The B19S strain has been found pathogenic for man [31]. The 19BA smooth strain used since 1946 by Vershilova [3] for human vaccination has been reported by Spink et al. [32] not to be safe enough. However, the use of this strain in cancer patients under clinical surveillance is considered by us as an acceptable risk. For human vaccination Vershilova has proposed the subcutaneous injection of 2.5×10^8 viable units, which induces agglutinins between Day 7 and Day 14 and reaction to

Melitin around Day 30 and Day 40. Zenkova [33] has recommended a further scarification by 2×10^9 organisms. In our clinical trials doses of 10^{10} organisms, i.e. 40 times the dose of the vaccine, were injected. In general this injection was tolerated well and no bacteremia was revealed by hemoculture. The evaluation of the invasiveness of the bacteria would be an important parameter to monitor in the treatment of tumours by live bacteria. However, no routine test is presently available. Needle biopsies have evidenced the presence of BCG in the liver after BCG scarification [34]. In the seven patients never submitted to chemo- or radiotherapy a clearcut increase in the blood mononuclear cell counts were observed.

The mechanisms by which live *Brucella* are effective against tumours is not completely understood. As with other intracellular bacteria or parasites (BCG, listeria, toxoplasma) a high level of macrophage activation is induced by committed T cells. This phenomenon, first described by Mackaness [35], has since been investigated by Riglar and Cheers [36]. The induction of type II interferon would be one aspect of that stimulation [29,37]. A high level of natural killer activity has also been observed by one of us many days after the ip injection in the mouse of live *Brucella* (in preparation). Such an effect has been previously reported with BCG [38].

Killed *Brucella*, even when capable of inducing specific immune responses, are probably not acting on the tumour through the same pathway. Specific and non-specific defense mechanisms against tumours have been found to be potentiated by inactivated bacteria or bacterial products: cytostatic or cytotoxic macrophages [39, 40], antibody-dependent cytotoxic lymphocytes [41, 42], T killer cells [43] and more recently NK cells [44,45]. Chirigos et al. [14] were able to demonstrate systemic immunity after the injection of Bru-pel and irradiated tumor cells.

The role played by T cells in the activation of the defense processes against tumours has been investigated by comparing normal and T-cell-deprived mice. The local injection of *Corynebacterium parvum* at the site of tumour implantation was found to be optimized by the presence of T cells [45]. These T-cells may have been useful to mount a specific response against the tumour. But it is more likely that they reacted against the bacterial antigens and contributed thus to produce an inflammatory reaction unfavourable for tumour growth [46]. When S- and R-inactivated *Brucella* were injected iv they affected differently cellular and antibody-mediated immune responses against SRBC. B19S organisms which displayed a strong surface antigenicity probably competed with SRBC antigens. This resulted in the diminution of the T-dependent DTH response against SRBC, a property not shared with B19R bacteria. As B19S and B19R influenced tumour growth in a roughly comparable manner it was concluded that the effect was not linked to an increase of T-dependent responses against the tumour. These results confirm those obtained with T cell-deprived mice in which the systemic injection of *C. parvum* is as active on thymectomized as in normal animals [47].

The increase of resistance against tumours in the first days following inoculation of killed *Brucella* does not seem to be related to spleen hypertrophy. Indeed, only strain B19S produced this effect, although B19S and B19R were comparably active on tumours. As has been reported [22], the increase of spleen weight is a haematological phenomenon linked to the migration of CFU from the bone marrow to the spleen. Its occurrence seems to depend on the presence of polysaccharides found on the surface of the S form of Gram negative bacteria and not of R. It has been shown that the synthesis of CSF induced by LPS is a property of the polysaccharide moiety [48]. The periodate oxidation of *C. parvum*, a treatment known to destroy carbohydrates, suppressed the ability of the organisms to provoke a spleen hypertrophy but did not alter the antineoplastic properties [49].

Among the hypotheses which have been proposed to explain the antitumour activity of microorganisms is their toxic effects. The first authors using bacterial products [50] observed hemorrhagic necrosis. The discovery that LPS induces tumor-necrotizing factor in animals which have received BCG [51] has re-emphasized this hypothesis. The chemical and biological properties of the endotoxins extracted from *B. abortus* are peculiar. The endotoxin of the S forms extracted by the Westphal method segregates in the phenolic phase and not in the aqueous phase, as is usual with Gram negative organisms. However, the endotoxin of R forms is present in the aqueous phase [52]. The endotoxin extracted has a low content in β-hydroxylated fatty acids and especially in β-hydroxymyristic acid, a substance characteristic of lipid A. The toxic properties of *Brucella* endotoxins are weaker than those of other Gram negative organisms. Quantities of *B. abortus* toxins 50 or 100 times more elevated than those of other Gram negative bacteria are necessary to induce comparable LD_{50} in mice or hyperthermic effects in rabbits (reviewed in ref. 53). However, when the whole S and R *Brucella* were compared to *Salmonella* for their toxicity the LD_{50} ranges were the same in normal mice but lower for *Brucella* in adrenalectomized mice. So the LPS would not be responsible for the whole toxicity. The reduction of the toxicity of *LPS* is known to be compatible with the antitumour effect [54], with the activation of macrophages [55] and with the tumour necrosis effect [56]. In the case of *B. abortus* two chemical treatments, ether and NaOH, and their sequential addition were found to diminish toxicity and preserve antitumour activity.

REFERENCES

1   Zourbas, J., Masse, L., Roussey, A., David, C., Morin, J. and Torte, J. Sampling survey and brucellosis among farmers and their families in Ille et Vilaine (Brittany). Int. J. Epidemiol. 6, 335, 1976.
2   Cotton, W.E., Buck, J.M. and Smith, H.E. Efficiency and safety of abortion vaccines prepared from *Brucella abortus* strains of different degrees of virulence. J. Agric. Res. 46, 291, 1976.
3   Vershilova, B.A. The use of live vaccine for vaccination of human beings against brucellosis in the USSR. Bull. WHO, 24, 85, 1961.
4   Hirnle, Z. The effect of *Brucella abortus* infection on transmissible Croker's sarcoma in mice. Acta Med. Pol. 1, 219, 1960.
5   Pilet, C. and Sabolovic, D. *Brucella abortus* et immunothérapie active non spécifique de la tumeur d'Erhlich. Bull. Ass. Franc. Vet. Microbiol. 7, 43, 1970.
6   Veskova, T.K., Chimishkyan, K.L., and Svet-Moldavsky, C.J. Effect of *Brucella abortus* vaccine (vaccine strain 19BA) on Rauscher leukemia virus and L 1210 leukemia in mice. J. Nat. Cancer Inst. 52, 1651, 1974.

14

7 De Santis, M. and Sega, E. The effect of living *Brucella abortus* vaccine in non-virus transplantable tumours. IRCS Med. Sci. 4, 261, 1976.

8 Chimishkyan, K.L., Belyanchikova, N.I., Kostrykina, V.N. and Nejland, E.N. Influence de *Brucella abortus* sur l'évolution de la leucose myéloïde aiguë chez la souris. Vopr Virusol SSSR 2, 202, 1977.

9 Dazord, L., le Garrec, Y., David, C. and Toujas, L. Resistance to transplanted cancer in mice increased by live *Brucella* vaccine. Br. J. Cancer 38, 464, 1978.

10 Dazord, L., le Garrec, Y., Bonnier, M. and Toujas, L. Increased resistance to tumor graft in mice injected by vaccinal strains of *Brucella abortus*. Rec. Res. Cancer Res. 75, 92, 1980.

11 Toujas, L., Sabolovic, D., Dazord, L., le Garrec, Y., Toujas, J.P., Guelfi, J. and Pilet, C. The mechanism of immunostimulation induced by inactivated *Brucella abortus*. Rev. Eur. Et. Clin. Biol. 17, 267, 1972.

12 Le Garrec, Y., Sabolovic, D., Toujas, L., Dazord, L., Guelfi, J. and Pilet, C. Activity of inactivated *Brucella* on murine tumors : prophylactic effect and combination with specific immunostimulation. Biomed. Exp. 21, 40, 1974.

13 Keleti, G., Feingold, D.S. and Youngner, J.S. Antitumor activity of a *Brucella abortus* preparation. Infect. Immun. 15, 846, 1977.

14 Chirigos, M.A., Stylos, W.A. and Schultz, R.M. Chemical and biological adjuvants capable of potentiating tumor cell vaccine. Cancer Res. 38, 1093, 1978.

15 Chirigos, M.A., Schultz, R.M., Pavlidis, N., Feingold, D.S. and Youngner, J.S. Comparative adjuvant effect of levamisole and *Brucella abortus* in murine leukemia. Cancer Treat. Rep. 62, 1943, 1970.

16 Schultz, R.M., Chirigos, M.A. and Pavlidis, N.A. Macrophage activation and antitumor activity of *Brucella abortus* ether extract, Bru-pel. Cancer Treat. Rep. 62, 1937, 1978.

17 Glasgow, L.A., Crane, J.L., Schleupner, C.J., Kern, E.R., Youngner, J.R. and Feingold, D.S. Enhancement of resistance to murine osteogenic sarcoma in vivo by an extract of *Brucella abortus* (bru-pel). Association with activation of reticuloendothelial system macrophages. Infect. Immun. 23, 19, 1979.

18 Fisher, B., and Gebhardt, M. Comparative effects of *Corynebacterium parvum*, *Brucella abortus* extract, *Bacillus Calmette Guerin*, Glucan, Levamisole and Tilorone with or without cyclophosphamide on tumor growth. Macrophage production and macrophage cytotoxicity in a murine mammary tumor model. Cancer Treat. Rep. 62, 1919, 1978.

19 Martin, A., Toujas, L., le Garrec, Y., Dazord, L. and Amice, J. Resistance to tumor graft in mice treated with inactivated *Brucella abortus* cultured in smooth or rough phase. J. Nat. Cancer Inst. 62, 123, 1979.

20 Le Garrec, Y., Martin, A., Collet, B., Toujas, L. and Pilet, C. Antitumor properties of chemically detoxified killed *Brucella abortus* organisms. Cancer Immunol. Immunother 11, 63, 1981.

21 Toujas, L., Dazord, L., and Guelfi, J. Increase of *Brucella*-induced immunostimulation by administration in combination with a specific antiserum. Rec. Results Cancer Res. 47, 302, 1974.

22 Toujas, L., Dazord, L., and Guelfi, J. Kinetics of proliferation of bone marrow cell lines after injection of immunostimulant bacteria. In: *Corynebacterium parvum* (B. Halpern Ed.), p. 117, 1975, Plenum; New York.

23 Le Garrec, Y., Toujas, L., Martin, A., Dazord, L. and Pilet, C. Influence of the antigenicity of *Brucella abortus* on the modification of the immune response to sheep erythrocytes. Infect. Immun. 20, 6, 1978.

24 Martin, A., le Garrec, Y., Dazord, L. and Toujas, L. Modulation of immune response by killed *Brucella abortus* organisms : comparison of the effects of smooth and rough strains on T-dependent responses. Infect. Immun. 21, 1027, 1978.

25 Dazord, L., Martin, A., le Garrec, Y. and Toujas, L. Resistance to peritoneal lymphoma graft induced by heat-killed S or R *Brucella abortus*. Cancer Immunol. Immunother. 38, 464. 1978.

26 Amice, J., Dazord, L. and Toujas, L. Generation of new macrophages after injection of killed *Brucella abortus* organisms. Cancer Immunol. Immunother. 4, 247, 1978.

27 Toujas, L., Collet, B., Dazord, L., le Garrec, Y. and David, C. Factors controlling the antitumor activity of *Brucella abortus*. INSERM Symposium series 97, 115, 1981.

28 Badakhsh, F.F. and Foster, J.W. Detoxification and immunogenic properties of endotoxin-containing precipitate of *Brucella abortus*. J. Bacteriol. 91, 494, 1966.

29 Youngner, J.S., Keleti, G. and Feingold, D.S. Antiviral activity of an ether extracted non viable preparation of *Brucella abortus*. Infect. Immun. 10, 1202 1974.

30 Raistrich, H., and Topley, W.W.C. Immunizing fractions isolated from Bac Aertrycke. Brit. J. Exp. Pathol. 15, 113, 1934.

31 Goret, P. and Pilet, C. La vaccination des bovins par le vaccin B19 et les vaccins semblables. Ann. Institut Pasteur 102, 774, 1962.

32 Spink, W.W., Hall, J.W., Finstau, J. and Mallet, E. Immunisation with viable *Brucella* organisms. Bull. WHO 26, 409, 1962.

33 Zenkova, N.F. Vaccination prophylactique par le vaccin brucellique vivant (méthode de scarification). Tr. Inst. Kraev. Pat. 3, 77, 1956.

34 Serrou, B., Michel, H., Dubois, J.B. and Serre, A. Hepatite granulomateuse par injection de BCG au cours de l'immunothérapie d'un mélanome malin. Biomed. Exp. 23, 236, 1975.

35 Mackaness, G.B. The immunological basis of acquired cellular resistance. J. Exp. Med. 120, 105, 1964.

36 Riglar, C. and Cheers, C. Macrophage activation during experimental murine brucellosis. II. Inhibition of in vitro lymphocyte proliferation by *Brucella*- activated macrophages. Cell. Immunol. 49, 154, 1980.

37 Bousquet-Ucla, C., Wietzerbin, J. and Falcoff, E. Studies on *Brucella* interferon : chromatographic behaviour and purification. Arch. Virol. 63, 57, 1980.

38 Wolfe, S.A., Tracey, D.E. and Henney, C.S. : Induction of natural killer cells by B.C.G. Nature 262, 584, 1976.

39 Hibbs, J.B., Lambert, L.J. and Remington, J.S. : possible role of macrophage-mediated cytotoxicity in tumor resistance. Nature (New Biol.) 235, 48, 1972.

40 Alexander, P. The functions of the macrophage in malignant disease. Ann. Res. Med. 27, 207, 1976.

41 Tagliabu, A., Mantovani, A., Polentarutti, N., Vecchi, A. and Streasico, S. Effect of immunomodulators on effector cells involved in antibody-dependent cellular cytotoxicity. J. Natl. Cancer Inst. 59, 1019, 1977.

42 Juy, D. and Leclerc, C. Enhancement of antibody dependent cell mediated cytotoxicity by an interphase material extracted from a non pathogenic strain of mycobacterium. Cancer Immunol. Immunother. 3, 23, 1977.

43 Fray, A., Crepin, Y., Platica, O., Sparros, L., Louvet, A. and Rabourdin, A. Action inhibitrice du Corynebacterium sur le développement des tumeurs malignes syngéniques et son mécanisme. C.R. Acad. Sci. Paris 276, 1911, 1973.

44 Herberman, R.B., Nunn, M.E. Holden, H.T., Staal, S. and Djeu, J.Y. Augmentation of natural cytotoxic reactivity of mouse lymphoïd cells against syngeneic and allogenic target cells. Internat. J. Cancer, 19, 555, 1977.

45 Scott, M.T. *Corynebacterium parvum* as a therapeutic antitumor agent in mice. II Local injection. J. Nat. Cancer Inst. 53, 861, 1974.

46 Tuttle, R.L. and North, R.J. Mechanisms of antitumor action of *C. parvum* : non-specific tumor cell destruction at site of immunologically mediated sensitivity reaction to *C. parvum*. J. Natl. Cancer Inst. 55, 1403, 1975.

47 Scott, M.T. *Corynebacterium parvum* as a therapeutic antitumor agent in mice. I. Systemic effect from intravenous injection. J. Natl. Cancer Inst. 53, 855, 1974.

48 Nowotny, A., Behling, U.H. and Chang, H.L. Relation of structure to function in bacterial endotoxins. J. Immunol. 115, 199, 1975.

49 Riveros-Moreno, V. and Niblock, A. Analysis of the effect of periodate oxydation and phenol extraction on the antitumour properties of *C. parvum*. Cancer Immunol, Immunother. 8, 265, 1980.

50 Coley, W.B. : Late results of the treatment of inoperable sarcoma by the mixed toxins of erysipelas and *Bacillus prodigiosus*. Am. J. Med. Sci. 131, 375, 1906.

51 Carswell, E.A., Old, L.J. Kassel, R.L., Greens, S., Fiore, N. and Williarson, B. An endotoxin-induced factor that causes necrosis of tumors. Proc. Nat. Acad. Sci. 73, 381, 1975.

16

52 Moreno, E., Pitt, M.W., Jones, L.M., Schurig, G.G. and Berman, D.T. Purification and characterization of smooth and rough lipopolysaccharides from *Brucella abortus*. Infect. Immun. 138, 361, 1979.

53 Moreno, E., Berman, D.T. and Boetcher, L.A. Biological activity of *Brucella abortus* polysaccharides. Infect. Immun. 31, 362, 1981.

54 Ribi, E., Parker, R. Strain, S.M., Mizano, Y., Nowotny, A., Von Eschen, K.B., Cantrell, J.L., McLaughlin, C.A., Hwang, K.M. and Goren, M.B. Peptides as requirement for immunotherapy of the guinea pig line 10 tumor with endotoxins. Cancer Immunol. Immunother. 7, 43, 1979.

55 Doe, W.F. and Henson, P.M. Macrophage stimulation by bacterial LPS. J. Exp. Med. 148, 544, 1978.

56 Nowotny, A., Golub S. and Key, B. Fate and effects of endotoxin derivatives in tumor bearing mice. Proc. Soc. Exp. Biol. Med. 136, 65, 1971.

CHAPTER 2

Antitumor activity of alkyllysophospholipids

P.G. Munder

Max-Planck-Institut für Immunbiologie, Freiburg i.Br. (FRG)

2.1. INTRODUCTION

Lysophospholipids are important intermediates in the biosynthesis and continuous renewal of phospholipids in cellular membranes of mammalian cells [1–4]. A cytotoxic concentration of these molecules is controlled by at least three enzymes and by their binding to lipoproteins and albumin, thus abolishing their potentially dangerous surface activity [1,4].

Besides their biochemical significance lysophospholipids exhibit in vivo a number of biological activities [5,6,7], some of them at extremely low concentrations [8,9]. Our studies on a biological role of lysophosphatidylcholine (LPC) was prompted by the observation that immunological adjuvants which have also been used in tumor therapy activate a phospholipase A after macrophages have been in contact with these compounds. The increased activity of this cellular enzyme causes a degradation of 3-*sn*-phosphatidylcholine (PC) and -ethanolamine (PE), accompanied by an increased formation of LPC [10,11,12]. Although LPC is in turn degraded to the non-toxic glycerophosphorylcholine (GPC), the phagocytes will finally be destroyed [11,12,13]. Using strong and persistent adjuvants like Freund's complete adjuvant, mycobacteria, silica, *Corynebacterium parvum* etc, this cytotoxic process causes the formation of granuloma in vivo and thereby apparently their efficacy in modifying immunological reactions. This process is also accompanied by an accumulation of LPC in vivo.

If endogenously formed LPC is considered to be a common denominator for the mechanism of adjuvants in vivo, exogenous LPC should then also act as an adjuvant. This was found to be true [12,14]. The short half-life of this molecule, however, apparently limited its biological efficacy [15,16]. It was therefore decided to synthesize derivatives of LPC theoretically with a much longer half-life and therefore a stronger and longer lasting immunobiological effect. These expectations were in part fulfilled. More important however, was the observation of an antitumor activity of some of the modified synthetic derivatives of the physiological LPC. Certain alkyllysophospholipids (ALP) have been found to activate host defense cells and the same molecules attack directly any of the tumor cells so far tested.

2.2 ALKYLLYSOPHOSPHOLIPIDS

Numerous modifications of physiological LPC are possible when lysophospholipids are synthesized. The synthesis, structure and physicochemistry of these compounds have been described elsewhere [17,18].

To obtain an optimal antitumor effect in vitro and in vivo two modifications are necessary.

1.   To prevent the degradation by lysophospholipases the aliphatic side chain has to be ether(alkyl) instead of ester(acyl) bonded.

2.   The OH-group in *sn*-2 has either to be omitted or blocked by methylation or benzylation to inhibit the acylation of the molecule to 3-*sn*-phosphatidylcholine. Figure 2.1 demonstrates the principal alterations.

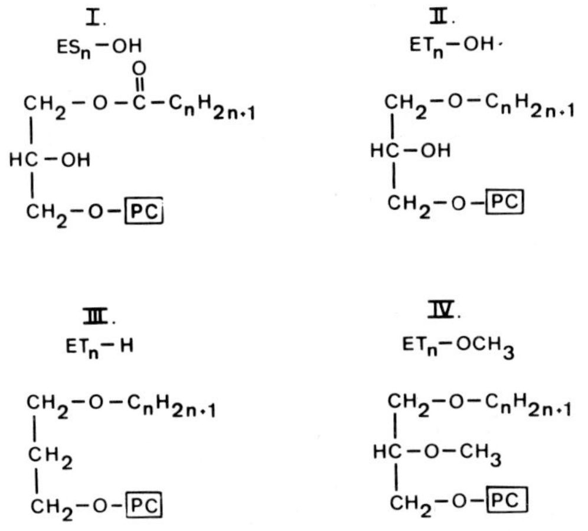

I.
ES_n-OH
$$CH_2-O-\overset{\overset{O}{\|}}{C}-C_nH_{2n\cdot1}$$
$HC-OH$
$CH_2-O-\boxed{PC}$

II.
$ET_n-OH\cdot$
$CH_2-O-C_nH_{2n\cdot1}$
$HC-OH$
$CH_2-O-\boxed{PC}$

III.
ET_n-H
$CH_2-O-C_nH_{2n\cdot1}$
CH_2
$CH_2-O-\boxed{PC}$

IV.
ET_n-OCH_3
$CH_2-O-C_nH_{2n\cdot1}$
$HC-O-CH_3$
$CH_2-O-\boxed{PC}$

Fig. 2.1. Chemical structure of different alkyl analogs (ALP) of LPC. The following abbreviated names will be used: ET stands for ether linkage of the aliphatic side chain, ES will denote ester derivatives; *n* gives the number of carbons per aliphatic chain and the following letters (H = hydrogen, OCH$_3$ = O-methyl, Benz = O-benzyl, OH = hydroxyl) give the chemical substitution of the C$_2$ of the glycerol backbone.

2.2.1. Antitumor activity in vivo

2.2.1.1. Ehrlich ascites tumor (EATC)
The EATC subline is highly malignant for NMRI mice. 10–100 cells will kill 100% of

the inoculated mice. When the ALPs were given ip prior to the tumor cells on day −30 to −4 almost, 100% of the animals survived the challenging injection of 1×10^4 EATC ip [19]. This confirms the results of others who found a similar protective antitumor effect with other immunomodulating substances and tumors [20]. This rather unspecific effect appears to be due to the accumulation of new host defense cells after the injection of an irritating agent into the peritoneal cavity. Further experiments, however, revealed a definite therapeutic effect when EATC were given ip and an ALP such as ET-18-OCH₃ daily iv, starting on day +1 to +9. Treatment beginning later was ineffective [19]. An intratumoral injection of 1–1000 μg ALP had no significant therapeutic effect, which seemed to indicate only a minor role for a direct cytotoxic effect of ALP on tumor cells in vivo.

As shown in Fig. 2.2 other ALPs are also effective, although to a lesser extent depending on the kind of modification.

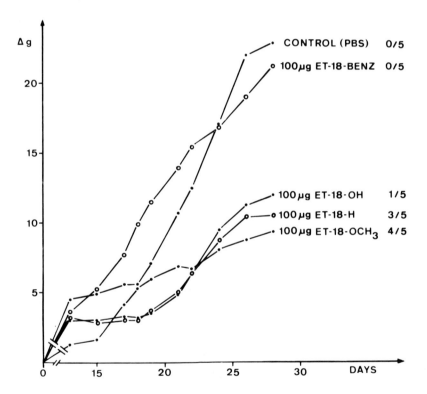

Fig. 2.2. Antitumor activity of various alkyl-lysophospholipids (ALP). NMRI mice were injected ip on day 0 with 1×10^4 EATC. Treatment was started on day +5 by giving the ALP iv for 16 days. Tumor growth was measured by weighing the mice twice weekly. The ordinate indicates the weight increase per mouse. SD was usually less than 5%.

ET-18-OCH₃ is the most effective compound, followed by ET-18-H and then by ET-18-OH, which can partially be metabolized. ET-18-Benz has always been ineffective for some as yet unknown reason. Perhaps the rather large benzyl group interferes with the interaction or uptake of the ALP into cellular membranes [21].

Table 2.1 summarizes the results of various experiments in which mice were inoculated with an increasing number of tumor cells and treated iv daily from day +7 to 28 with different concentrations of ET-18-OCH$_3$.

Table 2.I.

Influence of ET-18-OCH$_3$ (1–100 μg) on the ip growth of different inocula of EATC

Number of tumor cells	ET-18-OCH$_3$		
	1 μg*	10 μg	100 μg
1×10^4	3/5*	1/5	3/5
5×10^4	8/10	2/10	4/10
1×10^5	6/10	0/10	6/10
5×10^5	1/5	1/5	1/5

Control: Survivors/Total:0/30

Survivors were determined 4 weeks after the last mouse in the control group had died.

*NMRI mice were injected with ET-18-OCH$_3$ in 0.2 ml saline daily iv from day +7 to 28.

From these experiments the following conclusions can be drawn.

1. ET-18-OCH$_3$ inhibits tumor growth in concentrations as low as 1 μg per mouse per day.

2. Injection of ET-18-OCH$_3$ can cure part of the mice from a tumor load (1×10^5) more than a thousand-fold higher than the minimal killing dose ($10^1 - 10^2$ cells).

3. There is no apparent dose-response relationship, as 1 and 100 μg were equally effective, whereas 10 μg were much less active. Perhaps the induction or activation of ALP-metabolizing enzymes in the liver might interfere with a clear cut dose-response relationship. Pharmacokinetic studies should shed some light on this phenomenon.

2.2.2.2. MethA sarcoma

The growth of transplanted MethA sarcoma cells in (BALB/c × C57 Bl$_6$)F$_1$ mice is another tumor system in which the antitumor activity of various ALPs is extensively tested [19,22].

Table 2.2 demonstrates the antitumor activity of ET-18-OH, when given iv.1×10^5 MethA sarcoma cells were injected ic and treatment started on day +1 and +5, respectively, after implantation of the tumor cells.

Although other ALPs like ET-18-OCH$_3$ are also active in the MethA model, ET-18-OH has been superior in many experiments. Concentrations as low as 0.5 μg per mouse per day had a significant therapeutic effect when given iv, for 15–21 subsequent days. Lower concentrations were ineffective and doses higher than

Table 2.II.

Influence of ET-18-OH on the ic growth of MethA sarcoma

Treatment from day	ALP* (μg)	Mice with tumor on day:			
		8	14	21	28
+1	0	20	20	20	20
	10	8	8	5	3
	100	13	11	9	8
+5	10	18	16	11	9
	100	13	7	5	4

1×10^5 MethA sarcoma cells were implanted on day 0 in 0.2 ml saline.

*ET-18-OH was injected iv daily for 21 days.

100μg per mouse per day did not improve the results. Similar results could be obtained when the ALPs where given daily ic.

A decisive difference between alkyl- and acyllysophospholipids emerged when the compounds were given orally. Whereas substituted derivatives with an ester (acyl)-bonded aliphatic side chain (see Table 2.1) had slight effect when given iv or ic, their activity disappeared completely when given orally. Using this route of application only alkyllysophospholipids are able to inhibit the ic growth of the MethA sarcoma, as shown in Fig.2.3. Since these findings were made in most experiments ALPs are given orally.

2.2.2.3. 3-Lewis-Lung (3LL) carcinoma

This tumor has been used to study primarily the influence of ALPs on the development of metastases. The 3LL carcinoma spreads regularly from the primary inoculation site to the lung. Therefore, the effect of ALP on the primary as well as on the metastases could be studied [23].

Whereas doses between 10 and 50 μg/day per mouse of ET-18-OH or ET-18-OCH$_3$ seldom retarded the growth of the primary tumor (1×10^6 cells in the hind foot pad) and never cured an animal, higher doses (100–250 μg/day per mouse) inhibited it significantly. After amputation of the tumor-bearing leg, oral application of ALP stopped the development of metastases, leading to the survival of 40–60% of the treated mice as compared to none in the control [23].

2.2.2.4. Myelomas

MPC 11 in BALB/c and X5563 in C3Hf mice were likewise used as tumor models. Subcutaneous growth of both tumors could be retarded or inhibited provided the initial tumor growth did not exceed 5×10^5 cells/mouse. Again, oral application was at least as effective as iv, and better than sc or im treatment. Established tumors with a diameter of 0.8–1 cm regressed completely when the mice were treated for 2–3 weeks with 50–100 μg ALP [19].

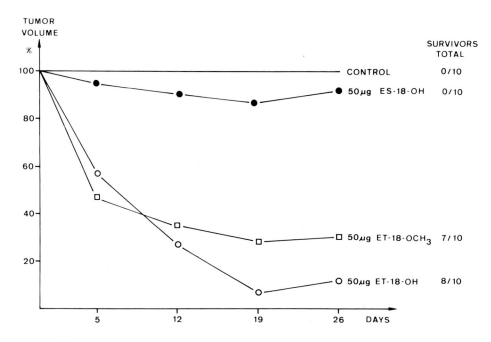

Fig. 2.3. Growth of Meth-A sarcoma during oral application of ALP. (BALB/c × C58 BL/6)F$_1$ mice were injected with 1×10^5 MethA sarcoma cells ic. The mice were fed daily with the lysophospholipids. Tumor volume was determined by measuring once per week two diameters of the growing tumors. The untreated control is set at 100%. After 4 weeks the tumor volume in the ten mice of the control group was usually 90–100 cm^3.

2.2.3. Antitumor activity in vitro

2.2.3.1. Elicitation of tumoricidal macrophages

Intraperitoneal injection of ALP induces a population of cells which inhibits the growth of syngeneic tumor cells in vivo. When these cells are removed from the peritoneal cavity and incubated in vitro with syngeneic tumor cells, DNA synthesis and cellular proliferation is almost completely stopped (see Fig. 2.4).

Cells obtained between days 3 and 6 after the injection of ALP have an optimal antitumor capacity, whereas cells collected only hours after the injection enhance the growth of tumor cells. Cells obtained after 10 days or later display a declining activity. These patterns are similar to the one observed after the injection of live BCG, *C. parvum*, FCA and other immunomodulators.

The elicitation of peritoneal exudate cells (PEC) by ALP is a rather unspecific phenomenon. However, the cells can be further activated in vitro when incubated with such ALPs as ET-18-OCH$_3$ and ET-18-H, but only poorly by ET-18-OH. Compounds containing an acyl bond are completely ineffective. Fig. 2.5. summarizes some of these results.

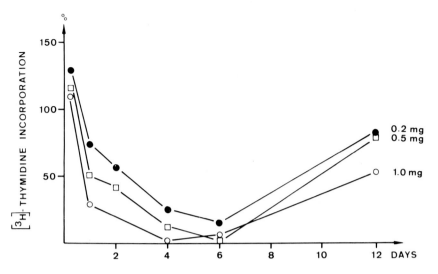

Fig. 2.4. Elicitation of tumorcidal peritoneal cells by ALP(ET-18-OCH$_3$). ALP was injected in 0.5 ml physiological saline. On the days indicated 3–5 mice were sacrificed and the PEC collected by rinsing the peritoneal cavity with 5 ml tissue culture medium (DMEM). The PEC were then incubated with target cells (MethA sarcoma) in a ratio of 10:1 and the [^{3}H]thymidine incorporation of the target cells measured after 24–48 h. The values are expressed as percentage incorporation of tumor cells in the presence of normal peritoneal cells.

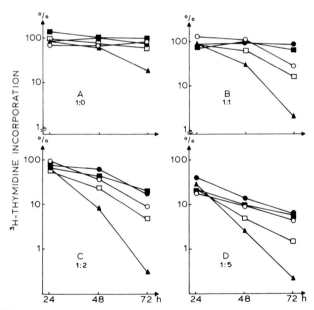

Fig.2.5. Activation of PEC by ALP in vitro. PEC were obtained as described (Fig. 2.4.). These cells were incubated with MethA sarcoma cells in the ratio 1:0(A), 1:1(B), 1:2(C) and 1:5(D) and 5µg of ALP. Total volume 5 ml (DMEM + 10% FCS). After 24,48 and 72 h, 1 ml of the cell suspension was withdrawn, placed into microtiter plates, washed and then pulsed with [^{3}H]thymidine. ▲ – ▲, ET-18-OCH$_3$; ■ – ■, ES-18-H; □ – □, ET-18-OH; ● – ●, control; ○ – ○, ET-18-H.

In these experiments the ALP were present during the entire period of effector: target cell interaction. This is, however, unnecessary. PEC can be incubated with 5–15 μg ET-18-OCH$_3$ for 24–48 hours, washed and then co-cultured with tumor cells. Under these experimental conditions the increase in tumorcidal activity is even greater as compared to the control PEC. If the active population is separated into adherent and nonadherent cells, only the former block tumor cell proliferation. This points to the macrophages as the most important cells mediating the antitumor effect of ALP. This assumption is supported by numerous studies in which 10–14 day old pure syngeneic bone marrow macrophages were used as effector cells. These macrophages are free from lymphocytes and granulocytes which might play a role when using PEC [24]. Normal bone marrow macrophages (BMM) have a slight antitumor effect which might depend on the batch of fetal calf serum used for cultivation. But after incubation with ALPs the tumor toxicity increases several fold [19]. The antitumor effect is already present at a ratio of 1:1 tumor cell:activated macrophages. In most experiments, [^{3}H]thymidine incorporation was used as a parameter for tumor cell proliferation after they had been in contact for 1–3 days with activated macrophages. This parameter was much more sensitive and reliable in our hands than the other methods measuring the release of isotopes from pre-labeled tumor cells. It should, however, be pointed out, that the cultivation system used allows the separation of the tumorcidal period from the time in which the label is incorporated [25,26,27]. Under these conditions, undamaged tumor cells will incorporate [^{3}H]thymidine, in the absence of unlabelled thymidine, which could be released from macrophages during the labeling pulse. Nevertheless, the actual number of tumor cells having grown in the absence of macrophages for a further 48 h has been determined in order to measure the regrowth capacity of the remaining cells and to correlate it with the labeling data. Over a wide range of tumor cell numbers both assays correlated well. Only with very high (10^6) or very low cell numbers (5×10^3 per ml) did cell counting prove to be more exact as determined by a calibration curve. Anyway, both assays proved beyond any doubt that ALP-activated macrophages are not only cytostatic but also cytotoxic. After 72 h only about $1–2 \times 10^4$ out of 5×10^5 tumor cells are alive in culture after having been incubated with activated macrophages in a ratio of 1:10.

As with PEC, BMM are more cytotoxic when preincubated with ALP (5–15 μg ml^{-1}) for at least 12 h. The prerequisites in the molecular structure for effective activation are again the alkyl bond and the substitution in *sn*-2. The length of the aliphatic side chain has also some influence, as derivatives with a chain length of 12 carbon atoms are either ineffective or have to be used in a 10-fold higher concentration. ALPs with a chain length of 20 or more carbon atoms are also inactive. Other modifications of the molecule are presently under investigation.

2.2.4. Direct cytotoxicity of ALP

While studying the mechanism by which tumoricidal macrophages are generated by ALP in vitro a direct cytotoxic effect of these activating substances on tumor cells

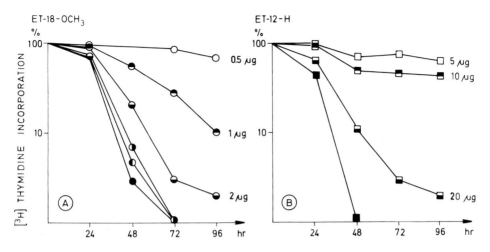

Fig. 2.6. Direct destruction of human leukemic cells by ALP. [^{3}H]thymidine incorporation into leukemic cells in the presence of increasing amounts of a short (ET-12-H) and a long chain ALP(ET-18-OCH$_3$). Quadruplicate cultures; SD = 2–5%.

was noted. This cytotoxicity was not due to the surface activity of this class of compounds mainly for the following reasons:

1.   The cytotoxicity developed within days as compared to minutes in a hemolytic reaction.

2.   All the substances used, including the acyllysophospholipids, have a similar surface activity but only substituted ALPs are cytotoxic for tumor cells.

3.   At the concentrations used (1–15 µg ml^{-1}) all lysophospholipids are bound to the proteins of the 10% serum in the medium. Immediate lysis occurs only above 50 µg ALP per ml.

A typical example of the course of the direct cell destruction by ALP is shown in Fig.2.6. in which human leukemic cells were incubated with two ALPs.

There is a clear relationship between the concentration of ET-18-OCH$_3$ and the inhibition of [^{3}H]thymidine incorporation. Morphologically, the cells swell during the first 24–48 h accompanied by an increased formation of multinucleated cells, which is then followed by complete lysis after 72–96 h. ET-12-H induces a similar pattern of cytolysis but at higher concentrations. The details of direct tumor cell destruction by ALP have been described extensively elsewhere [29]. More than a hundred freshly isolated or established human and animal tumor cells have been tested for their sensitivity towards cell destruction by ALP in vitro [26,28–34]. All these cells are destroyed except melanoma cells. Biochemically, the substituted ALP interfere with the phospholipid metabolism of tumor cells inhibiting essentially the synthesis of 3-*sn*-phosphatidylcholine. They are transferred from the lipoproteins of the serum to the lipid bilayer of the membranes and compete with the physiological 2-lysophosphatidylcholine in the continuous renewal of the phospholipid bilayer [30]. As the alkyl bond can only be split by the alkyl cleavage enzyme, which is not present or only at very low activity in tumor cells, the ALP molecules will accumulate in such cells and thus induce the process of cellular destruction.

2.2.5. Toxicology of ALP

Some preliminary toxicological studies have been performed using ET-18-OCH$_3$ in mice, rats, rabbits, baboon and vervet. In mice and rats the LD$_{50}$ was 55 mg kg^{-1} given iv. Usually, the animals died within 10–30 min. When given orally the LD$_{50}$ in mice was between 200 and 250 mg kg^{-1}. The mice died within 5–9 h after the body temperature has dropped to room temperature. Macroscopically no lesions in the gastro-intestinal tract were found. The histology after LD$_{50}$ iv or po has still to be examined. Doses below 40 mg kg^{-1} iv or below 150 mg kg^{-1} po are usually well tolerated even when given for several days. No hemolysis, hematuria, or hemoglobinuria was seen. There was no sign of liver or kidney damage except in animals that had received the LD$_{50}$ and survived. In these animals, urea levels rose slowly for several days and then declined to normal values.

In rabbits LD$_{50}$ was 4 mg kg^{-1}. The animals died within minutes. Respiratory stress was the first prominent pathological sign followed by severe cramps, then death. In this species, sudden death at this low dose might be due to a (PAF)-like activity [35]. Surprisingly, rabbits nevertheless tolerated up to 120 mg kg^{-1} ET-18-OCH$_3$ when given slowly (2–3 h) iv.

In baboons and vervets an LD$_{50}$ of 60 mg kg^{-1} was determined. If this dose was given rapidly in a rather small volume (20–50 ml in 5 min) immediate intravasal hemolysis occurred followed by hematuria and hemoglobinuria in 30–50 kg animals. If the volume/unit time was increased several times (up to 1000 ml over 1–2 h) these symptoms disappeared. Nevertheless, half of the baboons died after 60 mg kg^{-1}. At post mortem, the dead animals had enlarged kidneys. Other organs were macroscopically normal.

Vervets were treated 10 times for 3 weeks with 1 mg, 5 mg and 20 mg kg^{-1} ET-18-OCH$_3$. Urea, bilirubin, LDH, SGOT, SGPT, alkaline phosphatase, triglycerides and phospholipids and the important hematological values in peripheral blood were measured. There were no persistent pathological findings and none of the animals died due to the application of ALPs.

2.3. CONCLUSIONS

Among the lysophospholipids, substituted ALPs represent a class of compounds which possesses a unique property. In one and the same molecule two biological functions are combined which act synergistically in the defense against tumors.

1. ALPs induce in vivo and vitro the generation of tumoricidal macrophages, after these substances have been in contact with these host defense cells for several hours or days. They increase the tumoricidal capacity of macrophages several fold.

2. At the same time, the same 'activating' molecules exert a direct selective cytotoxic effect on tumor cells in the absence of any host defense cells. In this way they act like specific chemotherapeutics which affect the tumor cell membrane.

Both activities are clearly related to defined molecular structures of the substances.

Although many problems remain to be solved before a definite answer to this two-sided synergistic activity can be given the following preliminary explanations might be offered.

Whenever alkyllysophospholipids like ET-18-OH are adsorbed by tumor cells they can channel these compounds into the cellular phospholipid metabolism, provided the OH group is not substituted. The resulting 1-alkyl-2-acyl-phosphatidylcholine will be temporarily consistent with cellular survival as similar compounds are already present in tumor cells [36–39].

If, however, the ALP is substituted, as in ET-18-OCH$_3$, the molecule can neither be acylated nor degraded by cleavage of the alkyl bond. Tumor cells have no cleavage enzyme or only with very low activity [40,41]. Therefore, these ALPs will accumulate and induce a slow, progressive destruction of the tumor cell, forming actual 'holes' in the membrane which can be seen by scanning electron microscopy. When normal cells like macrophages adsorb substituted ALPs they can degrade the substituted molecules because they can cleave the alkyl bond as they have the required enzyme. This alkyl bond-splitting enzyme can even be activated by the addition of the substrate ALP to macrophages [29]. After close contact between tumor cell and ALP-activated macrophages, the activated enzyme of the effector cell might then also attack the alkyl bond of the cellular phospholipids in the tumor cell membrane. If at the same time tumor cells accumulate substituted ALPs the permeability barrier of the cell is weakened and the attack of the activated macrophage might act synergistically in killing the tumor cell. Moreover, even normal nonactivated macrophages are then able to kill tumor cells. Both mechanisms might act in vivo and in vitro.

It should, however, be pointed out that at least ET-18-OCH$_3$ has a chemical structure very close to the physiological compound described as platelet activating factor (PAF) [8,42]. It seems therefore possible that this biological activity also plays a role in tumor destruction, but only in vivo.

REFERENCES

1   Mulder, E., Van den Berg, J.W.O., and Van Deenen, L.L.M. Metabolism of red-cell lipids. II. Conversions of lysophosphoglycerides. Biochim. Biophys. Acta 106 118-127, 1965.
2   Hill, E.E., and Lands, W.E.M. Phospholipid Metabolism. in Lipid Metabolism (S.J. Walil Ed.), pp. 185-277, 1970, Academic Press Inc.; New York.
3   Ferber, E. Phospholipid dynamics in plasma membranes. in Biological Membranes (D. Chapman and D.F.H. Wallach Eds), pp. 221-252, 1973, Academic Press; New York.
4   Van den Bosch, H. Phosphoglyceride metabolism. Annu. Rev. Biochem. 43, 243. 1974.
5   Hung, S.C. and Melnykovych, G. Alkaline phosphatase in HeLa cells. Stimulation by phospholipase A$_2$ and lysophosphatidylcholine. Biochim. Biophys. Acta 429 409-420, 1976.
6   O'Doherty, P.J.A., Smith, N.B. and Kuksis, A. Stimulation of CDP-choline biosynthesis by enantiomeric lysophosphatidylcholines in rat intestinal mucosa. Arch. Biochem. Biophys. 180, 10-18, 1977.
7   Shier, W.T., Baldwin, J.H., Nilsen-Hamilton, M., Hamilton, R.T. and Thanassi, N.M. Regulation of guanylate and adenylate cyclase activities by lysolecithin. Proc. Natl. Acad. Sci. USA 73, 1586-1590, 1979.

8   Cusak, N.J. Platelet-activating factor. Nature 285, 10, 1980.
9   Pinckard, R.N., Halonen, M., Palmer, J.D., Butler, C., Shaw, J.O. and Henson, P.M. Intravascular aggregation and pulmonary sequestration of platelets during IgE-induced systemic anaphylaxis in the rabbit: Abrogation of lethal anaphylactic shock by platelet depletion. J. Immunol. 119, 2185-2193, 1977.
10 Munder, P.G. and Modolell, M. The influence of *Mycobacterium bovis* and *Corynebacterium parvum* on the phospholipid metabolism of macrophages. Recent Results Cancer Res. 47, 244-250, 1974.
11 Munder, P.G. and Lebert, St. The activation of phospholipase A in macrophages after the phagocytosis of silica and other cytotoxic dusts. in Inhaled Particles IV (W.H. Walton Ed.), pp. 531-541, 1977; Pergamon Press; Oxford.
12 Munder, P.G., Weltzien, H.U. and Modolell, M. Lysolecithin analogs: a new class of immunopotentiators. in Immunopathology (P.A. Miescher Ed.), pp 411-424, 1976, Schwabe & Co. Publishers; Basel.
13 Munder, P.G., Modolell, M., Ferber, E. and Fischer, H. The relationship between macrophages and adjuvant activity. in Mononuclear Phagocytes (R. van Furth, Ed.), pp. 445-460, 1970, Blackwell Scientific Publications; Oxford.
14 Munder, P.G., Modolell, M., Raetz, W. and Luckenbach, G.A. Primary antibody formation in vitro by mouse cells in a complete homologous system. Eur. J. Immunol. 3, 454-457, 1973.
15 Modolell, M., and Munder, P.G. The action of purified phospholipase B in inflammation and immunity. Int. Arch. Allergy 43, 724-739, 1972.
16 Munder, P.G., Ferber, E., Modolell, M. and Fischer, H. The influence of various adjuvants on the metabolism of phospholipids in macrophages. Internat. Arch. Allergy 36 117-128, 1969.
17 Eibl, H. and Westphal, O. Synthesen von Cholinphosphatiden. V. Palmitoylpropandiol(1,3)-phosphorylcholin(2-Desoxylysolecithin) und Alkandiol-Analoga. Ann. Chem. 709, 244-247, 1967.
18 Weltzien, H.U., Arnold, B. and Westphal, O. Synthesen von Cholinphosphatiden. IX. ^{14}C-markierte Lysolecithin Analoga. Ann.Chem. 1439-1444, 1973.
19 Munder, P.G., Modolell, M., Bausert, W., Oettgen, H.F. and Westphal, O. Alkyllysophospholipids in cancer therapy. in Augmenting Agents in Cancer Therapy (E.M. Hersh et al. Eds), pp. 441-458, 1981, Raven Press; New York.
20 Woodruff, M.F.A. The interaction of cancer and host, pp. 187-222, 1980, Grune & Stratton; New York.
21 Weltzien, H.U., Arnold, B. and Reuther, R. Quantitative studies on lysolecithin-mediated hemolysis. Use of ether-deoxy lysolecithin analogs with varying aliphatic chainlengths. Biochim. Biophys. Acta 466, 411-421, 1977.
22 Tarnowski, G.S., Mountain, I.M., Stock, C.C., Munder, P.G., Weltzien, H.U. and Westphal, O. Effect of lysolecithin and analogs on mouse ascites tumors. Cancer Res. 38, 339-344, 1978.
23 Berdel, W.E., Bausert, W.R., Weltzien, H.U., Modolell, M., Widmann, K.H. and Munder, P.G. The influence of alkyl-lysophospholipids and lysophospholipid activated macrophages on the development of metastasis of 3-Lewis lung carcinoma. Eur. J. Cancer 16, 1199-1204, 1980.
24 Metcalf, D. Hemopoietic colonies. Recent results in cancer research 61, 12-19, 1977, Springer Verlag; Berlin.
25 Munder, P.G., Modolell, M. and Wallach, D.F.H. Cell propagation of polymeric fluorocarbon as a means to regulate pericellular pH and pO_2 in cultured monolayers. FEBS Lett. 15, 191-196, 1971.
26 Berdel, W., Fink, U., Egger, B., Reichert, A., Munder, P.G. and Rastetter, J. Growth inhibition of malignant hypernephroma cells by autologous lysophospholipid incubated macrophages obtained by a new method. Anticancer Res. 1, 135-140, 1981.
27 Van der Meer, J.W.M., Bulterman, D., van Zwet, T.L., Elzenga-Claasen, J. and van Furth, R. Culture of mononuclear phagocytes on a teflon surface to prevent adherence. J. Exp. Med 147, 271-276, 1978.
28 Berdel, W., Fink, U., Egger, B., Reichert, A., Munder, P.G. and Rastetter, J. Inhibition by alkyl-lysophospholipids of tritiated thymidine uptake in cells of human malignant urologic tumors. J. Natl. Cancer Inst. 66, 813-817, 1981.

29 Andreesen, R., Modolell, M., Weltzien, H.U., Eibl, H., Common, H.H., Löhr, G.W. and Munder, P.G. Selective destruction of human leukemic cells by alkyl-lysophospholipids. Cancer Res. 38, 3894-3899, 1978.

30 Modolell, M., Andreesen, R., Pahlke, W., Brugger, U. and Munder, P.G. Disturbance of phospholipid metabolism during the selective destruction of tumor cells induced by alkyl-lysophospholipids. Cancer Res. 39, 4681-4686, 1979.

31 Maistry, L., Robinson, K.M., Evers, P., Munder, P.G. and Andreesen, R. Morphological effects of an antitumor agent on human esophageal carcinoma cells. Scanning Electron Microscopy III, 109-114, 1980.

32 Runge, M., Andreesen, R., Pfleiderer, E. and Munder, P.G. Destruction of human solid tumors by alkyl-lysophospholipids. J. Natl. Cancer Inst. 64, 1301-1306, 1980.

33 Andreesen, R., Modolell, M. and Munder, P.G. Selective sensitivity of chronic myelogenous leukemia cell populations to alkyl-lysophospholipids. Blood 54, 519-523, 1979.

34 Westphal, O., Westphal, U., Andreesen, R. and Munder, P.G. Anti-tumor effects of bacterial endotoxin (lipopolysaccharides, lipid A) and synthetic lysolecithin analogues. Pontificiae Academiae Scientiarum Scripta Varia 43, 323-354, 1979.

35 Henson, P.M. and Pinckard, R.N. Basophil-derived platelet-activating factor (PAF) as an in vivo mediator of acute allergic reactions: demonstration of specific desensitization of platelets to PAF during IgE-induced anaphylaxis in the rabbit. J. Immunol. 119, 2179-2184, 1977.

36 Waku, K., Uda, Y. and Nakazawa, A. Lipid composition in rabbit sarcoplasmic reticulum and occurrence of alkyl ether phospholipids. J. Biochem. (Tokyo) 69, 483-491, 1971.

37 Mangold, H.K. Biological effects and biomedical applications of alkoxylipids. in Ether Lipids (F. Snyder Ed.), pp. 157-176, 1972; Academic Press, New York.

38 Wood, R. and Snyder, F. Characterization and identification of glyceryl ether diesters present in tumor cells. J. Lipid Res. 8, 494-500, 1967.

39 Snyder, F. Ether-linked lipids and fatty alcohol precursors in neoplasms. in Ether Lipids, Chemistry and Biology (F. Snyder Ed.), pp. 273-296, 1972, Academic Press, New York.

40 Soodsma, J.F., Piantadosi, C. and Snyder, F. Partial characterization of the alkylglycerol cleavage enzyme system of rat liver. J. Biol. Chem. 247, 3923-3929, 1972.

41 Soodsma, J.F., Piantadosi, C. and Snyder, F. The biocleavage of alkyl glyceryl ethers in Morris hepatomas and other transplantable neoplasms. Cancer Res. 30, 309-311, 1970.

42 Hanahan, D.J., Munder, P.G., Satouchi, K., McManus, M. and Pinckard, R.N. Potent platelet stimulating activity of enantiomers of acetyl glyceryl ether phosphorylcholine and its methoxy analogues. Biochem. Biphys. Res. Commun. 99, 183-188, 1981.

CHAPTER 3

Experimental and clinical studies with OK-432

A streptococcal preparation with immunomodulating properties

M. Micksche[a], E.M. Kokoschka[b], T. Luger[b], H. Rainer[c], C. Dittrich[c], K. Moser[c], R. Jakesz[d], A. Fritsch[d], T. Hoshino[e], M. Al-Hashimi[a], S. Yamagata[a], M. Colot[a] and A. Uchida[a]

[a] *Institute for Cancer Research;* [b] *II. Department of Dermatology;* [c] *Clinic for Chemotherapy, Department for Oncology:* [d] *I. Department of Surgery; University of Vienna, Borschkegasse 8a, A-1090 Vienna (Austria); and II. Medical Clinic, Department of Medicine, Medical Faculty, Kyoto University (Japan)*

SUMMARY

OK-432, a streptococcal preparation, has been developed by Okamoto in Japan. Several animal studies have documented the tumor growth-inhibiting and immunomodulating properties of this agent.

In cancer patients immune modulation has also been documented after OK-432 therapy, resulting in an increase of lymphocyte blastogenic response to mitogens, normalization of the lymphocyte subpopulation's constitution and, furthermore, reduction in the activity of suppressor cells. Additionally, a therapeutic effect has been described in adjuvant therapy trials in both lung and gastric cancer.

We have investigated the influence of OK-432 on NK-cell activity in mice and found especially that the iv route enhances natural killing of splenocytes.

In a Lewis lung tumor system, iv application of several doses of OK-432 significantly inhibited the formation of pulmonary metastases.

Our time lapse studies on human malignant melanoma cells incubated with OK-432 in vitro give some further confirmation that OK-432 has a direct cytostatic activity on tumor cells.

In vitro incubation of patients' mononuclear peripheral blood leukocytes with OK-432 revealed that this preparation is able to enhance killing against the natural killer cell-sensitive line K-562.

A Phase I study using several doses of OK-432 given by a variety of routes (iv, im, id, it, ip) in patients with advanced solid malignancies showed that OK-432 can be applied safely and without severe side effects.

Besides this, in some patients – especially in cases of malignant melanoma – a beneficial clinical outcome has been noted. Furthermore, we have evidence from these investigations that OK-432 therapy enhances lymphocyte blastogenic response to mitogens and also natural killer cell activity.

In a randomized trial, where patients with radically operated gastric cancer are receiving no further therapy (group A), chemotherapy (group B) and immuno-(OK-432)-chemotherapy (group C), no significant differences in relapse rate between the three therapy arms have been noted so far.

From the present studies we can conclude that OK-432 is a potent immune-modulating agent in both animal models and cancer patients and possesses therapeutic efficacy.

3.1. INTRODUCTION

Immunotherapy of cancer has not yet reached routine clinical application, although there is an increasing number of trials showing positive clinical effects in prolonging both disease-free intervals and survival times [22]. The major aim of immunother-apy is to restore the immune functions of patients who are immunodepressed due to malignant disease or reduce the side effects resulting from cytoreductive therapy. Immune modulators that are at present being investigated in experimental and clinical studies include bacterial and mammalian products [2,35], as well as synthetic agents [14]. Although some progress is evident, further screening for such products, recently designated as 'biologic response modifiers', and also further immunopharmacologic studies on the mechanisms underlying the recognized immune modulation, are required [2].

One attempt along this line is the use of streptococcal preparations for cancer therapy. Following Bush's observation of tumor regressions in patients with erysipelas infections, Coley developed a bacterial extract for treatment of cancer patients and reported a beneficial therapeutic effect [4,27]. Animal studies giving good evidence of the possible therapeutical efficacy of hemolytic streptococci were performed in the 1960s, but were not continued to the stage of clinical use [9].

In 1966, Okamoto discovered that the cytostatic effect of β-hemolytic streptococ-ci on Ehrlich ascites carcinoma was greatly enhanced by treatment of the bacteria with penicillin followed by heating at 45°C. The cells thus treated lost the ability of causing infection and of producing streptolysin O and S [28]. The lyophilized form of this preparation, OK-432, was also found to be effective against various rat and mice ascites or solid tumors [8,20,44].

Furthermore, Aoki found that OK-432 therapy had immunoprophylactic and immunotherapeutic effects on leukemia in AKR mice. Treatment of animals for their life span with OK-432 resulted in a delay or even a reduction of leukemia incidence [1]. Some mechanisms responsible for the anticancer effect of OK-432 have been already described. According to these investigations, OK-432 has a direct cytocidal effect on tumor cells [30,33]. Furthermore, this agent displays immune modulating effects when applied intradermally, intramuscularly or intravenously to the host. The effects on immune function so far described include increases of antibody response and activation of macrophages and especially of

T-lymphocytes in animals [13,29,32,39].

One further interesting aspect is the induction of immune interferon by OK-432, as demonstrated in mice by Matsubara [23]. This stimulation of interferon production might be one additional mechanism that the immune modulating and therapeutic efficacy of OK-432 is based upon.

In cancer patients, immune modulation by OK-432 has also been documented, i.e. enhancement of delayed cutaneous hypersensitivity reactions, increase of circulating lymphocyte counts and normalization of the lymphocyte subpopulation constitution, enhancement of proliferative responses of lymphocytes to mitogens and, recently, a reduction of suppressor cells for mitogen response was demonstrated in patients after OK-432 therapy [24,36,37].

Besides the immune-restoring effect, therapy studies performed with OK-432 in Japan have demonstrated that this preparation is effective alone or in combination with chemotherapy for increasing the disease-free interval and survival time in adjuvant and palliative therapy studies, respectively [7,15,26,40].

Our investigations were performed in order to clarify the following questions:

(1) Has OK-432 an effect on natural killer (NK) activity in normal mice?
(2) Has OK-432 a therapeutic effect in Lewis lung tumor-bearing mice?
(3) Does OK-432 have cytostatic activity on in vitro cell cultures?
(4) Does OK-432 modify the cytotoxic cells of peripheral blood of cancer patients?
(5) Does OK-432 therapy modify the NK cell activity of treated patients?
(6) Is OK-432 tolerable for cancer patients (phase I study)?
(7) Is OK-432 effective in gastric cancer when combined with an adjuvant chemotherapy regimen?

3.2. PHARMACEUTICAL PREPARATION OF OK-432

OK-432 was supplied by Chugai Co., Japan [3] (via Casella Pharma, FRG) in vials containing lyophilized organisms. This pharmaceutical preparation is standardized by a variety of tests and a unit of 'KE' (= Klinische Einheit) is used to express the strength of the preparation. One KE corresponds to 0.1 mg dried streptococci. OK-432 is biologically lacking growth capacity both in vivo and in vitro, and devoid of streptolysin-O and -S production. Vials supplied contain 0.2, 0.5, 1 or 5 KE for clinical, and 50 KE for animal studies. The preparation was reconstituted with respective volumes of saline, according to the application site, immediately before administration.

3.3. EXPERIMENTAL STUDIES

3.3.1. Influence of OK-432 on NK-cell activity in mice

To investigate the influence of one single dose of OK-432 on NK-cell activity in mice (C57 BL/6J, BDF$_1$ hybrids), each group of 5–8 animals received 100 KE kg^{-1} of OK-432 iv or ip 36–48 h before preparation of spleen cells.

For kinetic studies of the influence of OK-432 on NK-cell activity animals were injected with single doses of 100 KE kg^{-1} iv on day -1, $-1\frac{1}{2}$, -2, -3, -5 and -7 before performing the assay. All animals were killed on day 0, and results compared with those of the group receiving no therapy.

A spleen weight index was also determined (spleen weight/body weight in g) on the respective experimental days.

3.3.1.1. NK assay

A 4-h, chromium-release assay was used to evaluate NK cell killing. Spleen cells were separated by Ficoll Hypaque centrifugation and resuspended in minimal essential medium (MEM) (Gibco Biocult) supplemented with 10% fetal calf serum (FCS) (Gibco Biocult). Target cells, YAC-1 (a Moloney leukemia virus-induced T-lymphoma, kindly supplied by G. Klein, Karolinska Institutet) and LLB (a continuous monolayer cell line established from Lewis lung tumor by Dr Vetterlein at our institute) were labelled with radioactive sodium chromate (^{51}Cr, Radiochemical Centre, Amersham, UK), and assay was performed at E:T (effector:target cells) ratios of 50:1, 100:1, 200:1, as described previously [5]. Results were expressed as percentage of specific release for each individual (for quadruplicate samples) by the formula:

$$\% \ ^{51}CR \ \text{release} = \frac{\text{Test cpm} - \text{spontaneous cpm}}{\text{Max cpm} - \text{spontaneous cpm}} \times 100$$

Statistical analysis was performed by Student's t-test.

3.3.1.1a. Influence of different routes (Table 3.I). Iv injection of OK-432 led to a significant increase in the percentage of specific cytotoxicity against YAC-1 and LLB in comparison to untreated control mice. Hybrid animals also developed increased cytotoxicity, after OK-432, against the LLB line. No significant change of spleen cell cytotoxicity was found after ip injection.

Table 3.I.

Influence of OK-432 on NK cell activity

OK-432	Cytotoxicity (different target lines) (%)		
	YAC-1[a]	LLB[a]	LLB[b]
No	21.2	12.7	8.3
iv	28.1*	18.1*	14.8*
ip	19.1	11.8	5.5

[a] C57 Bl.   [b] DBF$_1$.   *$P < 0.05$ (Student's t-test)

Spleen weight index was also found significantly increased in animals receiving OK-432 by the iv route, but not after ip administration (Table 3.II).

Table 3.II.

Influence of OK-432 on spleen weight (index)

OK-432	Spleen weight (index) of mice after OK-432		
	C57BL	C57BL	BDF$_1$
No	6.8±0.1	5.9±0.2	6.0±0.6
	(100)	(100)	(100)
iv	9.2±0.5	8.2±0.4	8.1±0.6
	(135)**	(139)**	(134)*
ip	6.2±0.1	6.4±0.4	6.6±1.7
	(92)	(108)	(109)

*$P<0.001$.   **$P<0.01$.

3.3.1.2b. Kinetics of NK-cell activity after one single iv injection of OK-432 (Fig. 3.1). OK-432 was administered at a single dose of 100 KE kg^{-1}, on day 1, 1½, 2, 3, 5, or 7 before the assay was performed. NK-cell activity was found to be significantly ($P< 0.001$) increased by 24 h, reaching a peak by 36 h. After 2 days, reactivity returned to the normal level, and a decrease was found on days 5 and 7. Spleen weight index was highest 2 days after OK-432 application, declined by day 3 and 5, and increased again by day 6 (Fig. 3.1).

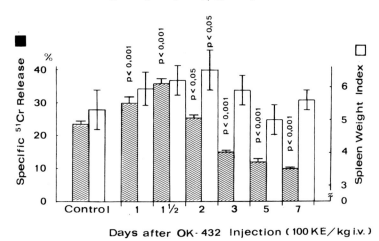

Fig. 3.1. Kinetics of NK cell activity after one single iv injection of OK-432. ■, specific chromium release (%); □, spleen weight index.

3.3.2. Influence of OK-432 on Lewis lung tumor

From Lewis lung tumor (LLT) maintained by serial transplantation in C57 BL /6J mice, a single cell suspension was prepared and 5×10^5 viable tumor cells were injected intramuscularly into the right hind thigh [18].

A dose of 50 KE kg^{-1} was injected iv for 7, and ip for 14 consecutive days, starting one day after inoculation of LLT. Ten animals per group were used, receiving iv OK-432 or saline and ip OK-432 or saline.

The tumor nodules were measured with a micrometer calliper on days 10, 14, 18, and 21 as described previously [17]. Mice were killed on day 21, lungs were removed surgically and fixed in Bouin's solution, and metastases were counted [17].

No significant differences were found in the primary tumor growth in iv saline and iv OK-432-treated mice. Mice receiving OK-432 ip showed a significant inhibition of tumor growth in comparison to animals receiving saline ip (Table 3.III).

Iv administration of OK-432 led to a significant suppression of lung metastasis formation in comparison to saline-injected animals, whereas the ip route of OK-432 did not influence the formation of lung metastases (Table 3.IV).

Table 3.III.

Influence of OK-432 on primary tumor growth (LLT)

Day[a]	iv Route[b]		ip Route[c]	
	OK-432	Saline	OK-432	Saline
10	1.59±0.13*	1.86±0.27	1.50±0.52	1.81±0.19
12	2.15±0.18	2.46±0.24	1.93±0.57	2.35±0.25
14	2.91±0.39	3.10±0.29	2.56±0.58**	3.34±0.27
18	3.82±0.51	4.39±0.57	3.80±0.81	4.62±0.45
21	4.77±0.52	5.11±0.47	4.33±0.422***	5.46±0.143

Statistical analysis: Student's t-test: comparison was made between OK-432 and saline-injected animals (mean volume ± S.D.). * $P < 0.05$; ** $P < 0.01$; *** $P < 0.001$. Tumor measurement (volume) $V = 0.4$ $(a.b)$ cm^3. a and b are two perpendicular diameters.

[a] Day after tumor inoculation.
[b] Animals received for 7 consecutive days injections of OK-432 (100 mg/kg^{-1}) or saline, iv.
[c] Animals received for 14 consecutive days injections of OK-432 (100 mg/kg^{-1}) or saline, iv.

Table 3.IV.

Influence of OK-432 on number of metastases (LLT)

Route	OK-432	Saline	t-Test
iv	16.1±10.3	102.6±40.5	$P<0.001$
ip	79.6±90.0	98.8±76.5	n.s.

Mean no. of metastases ± S.D.; n.s. : not significant. Animals were sacrificed on day 21 after tumor inoculation.

3.3.3. In vitro effects of OK-432 on tumor cells

It has been already reported in animal tumor systems and also in clinical studies that when OK-432 is brought into direct contact with tumor cells (in vitro

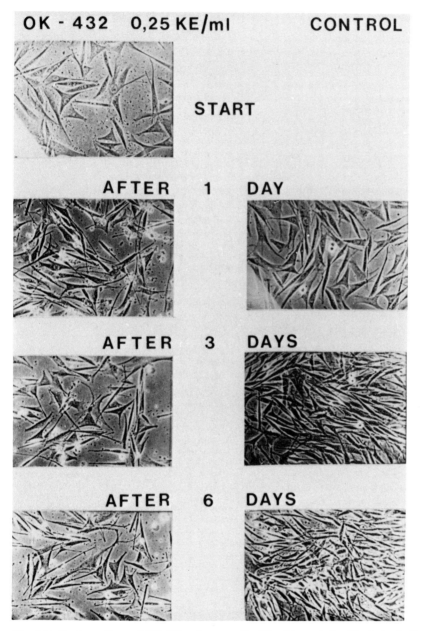

Fig. 3.2. In vitro effects of OK-432 on human cells. Microkinematographic study of effects of OK-43 on human malignant melanoma.

incubation or intralesional injection), this preparation has a direct cytostatic effect [8,30,33].

To investigate these properties, human melanoma cells cultured in vitro for several passages were explanted into Petri dishes and after overnight incubation the streptococcus preparation was added at a concentration of 0.25 KE ml^{-1}. Time lapse cinematography was used to document the effect of this preparation on tumor cell growth. During the observation period of 6 days OK-432 led to an inhibition of tumor cell multiplication, whereas control cultures displayed high mitotic activity, and a confluent monolayer was observed after this period in these cultures (Fig. 3.2).

Further studies are needed in order to investigate the growth-inhibiting effect of OK-432 on tumor cells in vitro. This inhibitory effect might have some implication for local immunotherapy with OK-432.

3.3.4. In vitro effects of OK-432 on cytotoxic cells of human peripheral blood

This part of the investigation was designed to evaluate the effect of OK-432 on the NK activity of human peripheral blood lymphocytes.

3.3.4.1. Cytotoxic assay
Peripheral blood lymphocytes were isolated from heparinized peripheral blood of patients with malignant melanoma and individuals without evidence of malignant disease by Ficoll-gradient centrifugation [37]. ^{51}Cr-labelled K-562 cells (an erythroleukemia cell line kindly provided by Dr Klein) were used as target cells. Effector cells were added to target cells at E:T ratios of 10:1, 20:1, 40:1, and mixtures were incubated for 4 h as described previously [25,38].

3.3.4.2. Dose response
Blood lymphocytes were incubated with varying concentrations of OK-432 for 20 h then washed and tested for cytotoxic activity.

The maximum enhancement of cytotoxic activity was observed when lymphocytes were incubated with a dose of 0.5 KE ml^{-1} for 20 h. However, in some cases 1×10^{-4} KE ml^{-1} of OK-432 significantly increased the activity (E:T 20:1). A representative experiment is shown in Fig. 3.3.

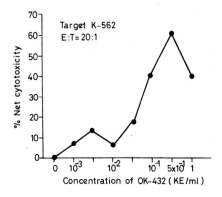

Fig. 3.3. Dose response of OK-432 on NK killing in vitro.

3.3.4.3. Influence of OK-432 on tumor effector cell viability

OK-432 has been demonstrated to have direct cytostatic and cytotoxic effect on tumor cells. In order to exclude the possibility that the increased cytotoxic activity measured may be attributed to a direct cytotoxic effect of OK-432, the effects of OK-432 on both effector and target cells were examined with a dose of 0.5 KE ml^{-1}.

Recovery of viable effector cells (trypan blue exclusion test) after 24 h incubation with OK-432 was comparable with that of lymphocytes incubated with medium alone, i.e. 87 ± 3% and 89 ± 3%, respectively.

K-562 target cells were also not affected by OK-432 (0.5 KE ml^{-1}) during a 4-h incubation period, as the percentage of released chromium was 6 ± 2% with medium and 7 ± 2% with OK-432. These results suggest that the augmented cytotoxic activity may be attributed to cytotoxic cells activated by OK-432.

3.3.4.4. Effect of OK-432 on NK-killing, different E:T ratios and comparison with IFN

Lymphocytes obtained from cancer patients were incubated with 0.5 KE ml^{-1} OK-432 or with Hu-IFN-α (human leukocyte interferon, α type obtained from Immunoski Zavod, Zagreb, Yugoslavia; specific activity 2.0×10^6 reference units per mg protein) at a concentration of 500 IU ml^{-1}. Untreated lymphocytes were used as controls. After 20 h incubation effector cells were washed, resuspended in medium and added to prelabelled target cells.

OK-432-activated cells augmented cytotoxic activity against K-562 at every effector to target cell ratio. Activation with OK-432 was comparable to that with interferon (Fig. 3.4).

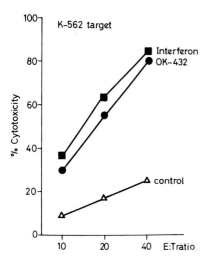

Fig. 3.4. Effect of OK-432 on NK killing. Different E:T ratios and comparison with interferon (Hu-IFN-α).

From these results it may be concluded that incubation of lymphocytes with OK-432 is able to activate or induce cytotoxic cells.

3.3.4.5. Influence of temperature on OK-432-induced cytotoxicity

To determine whether the activation of lymphocytes with OK-432 is dependent on cell metabolism, lymphocytes were incubated with OK-432 for 20 h at either 37°C or 4°C, and compared with the corresponding control lymphocytes. The cytotoxic activity of lymphocytes incubated with OK-432 at 37°C was significantly higher than that of the control lymphocytes. The lymphocytes incubated at 4°C did not show such increase (Fig. 3.5.). From this study it is evident that active cell metabolism is required for activation of cytotoxic cells.

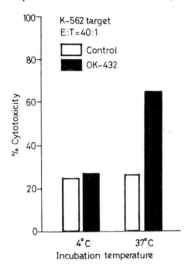

Fig. 3.5. Influence of temperature on OK-432-mediated cytotoxicity.

3.3.4.6. Influence of DNA synthesis

To ascertain whether the manifestation of enhanced cytotoxic activity with OK-432 requires a stage of DNA synthesis in the lymphocytes, lymphocytes were first treated with mitomycin C for 30 min, then washed and incubated with OK-432 for 20 h. The treatment increased the capacity of both mitomycin C-treated and untreated lymphocytes to lyse K-562 target cells (Fig. 3.6.). The results suggest that DNA synthesis of the lymphocytes is not necessary for augmentation of cytotoxic activity.

3.3.4.7. Cell population studies

OK-432 has been shown to activate macrophages in mice [13]. To check whether the augmented cytotoxic activity is mediated by activated monocytes or whether these cells are required for enhancement of cytotoxic activity, mononuclear cells were passed through a Sephadex G-10 column to remove monocytes, then incubated with OK-432. OK-432 enhanced the activity of both unseparated and monocyte-depleted lymphocytes (Fig. 3.7). The results suggest that the presence of monocytes is not necessary for the manifestation of augmented cytotoxic activity.

In order to distinguish which cell population is activated by OK-432 to cytotoxicity, monocyte-depleted pure lymphocytes were separated on a nylon wool column [37]. Nylon wool nonadherent cells of cancer patients showed depressed

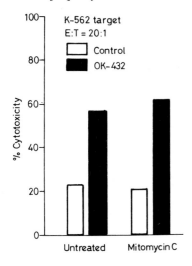

Fig. 3.6. Influence of DNA synthesis on OK-432-induced cytotoxicity.

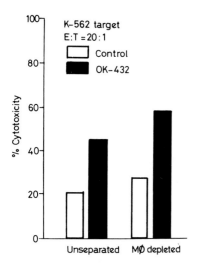

Fig. 3.7. Cell population studies. Influence of macrophage depletion on OK-432 enhancement of cytotoxicity.

but significant levels of NK activity, whereas nylon wool adherent cells showed no activity. After OK-432 treatment both nylon wool nonadherent and adherent cells showed significant increases in cytotoxic activity and no differences were observed between the activities of nylon wool nonadherent and adherent cells (Fig. 3.8).

The results suggest that OK-432 may not only enhance the cytotoxic activity of preexisting NK cells but also induce cytotoxic cells, perhaps from precursor cells.

These in vitro studies give evidence that OK-432 is able to enhance cytotoxic activity in separated and nonseparated, nylon wool adherent and nonadherent cell populations of peripheral blood. Further studies should clarify the cell type(s) responding to OK-432 in vitro activation.

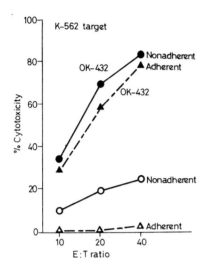

Fig. 3.8. Cell population studies. Adherent and nonadherent cells and cytotoxic activity after OK-432 incubation.

3.4. CLINICAL STUDIES

3.4.1. Influence of different routes of OK-432 application in vivo on NK-cell activity

For clinical application of OK-432 it seems to be important to prove that OK-432 therapy also enhances NK-cell activity and to know which route of administration of OK-432 is most effective for this purpose in cancer patients. Six patients with advanced malignant melanoma were treated with intravenous, intradermal or intramuscular single injections of OK-432 (1 KE) on day 0, and NK activity was monitored on days 0, 1, 2, 3 and 7. Control patients were not given any anticancer agents. Before therapy all patients showed impaired NK activity. To evaluate exactly the effects of OK-432 on NK activity, the change in cytotoxicity activity was calculated by subtracting pretreatment values from posttreatment values and standardized by control patients and normal controls. Fig. 3.8 shows the mean ± S.E. of 2 patients in each group. Iv and id single injections of OK-432 significantly enhanced NK activity, whereas im injections did not ($P < 0.01$, Student's t-test) (Fig. 3.9).

NK activity rapidly increased after a single dose of OK-432 and peaked on day 3, then decreased to pretreatment levels within 7 days (Fig. 3.9). The results suggest that iv and id injections of OK-432 are capable of enhancing NK activity but the enhancing effect soon disappears. Therefore, repeated iv or id injections of OK-432 may be necessary for maintaining augmented NK activity, and for im injection to induce the increase of cytotoxicity.

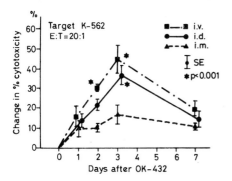

Fig. 3.9. Influence of different routes of OK-432 application in vivo on NK-cell activity.

3.4.2. Phase I study

Clinical reports from Japan have demonstrated that the OK-432 preparation can be safely given to patients. They gave further evidence that along with an immune modulation some benefit for the clinical outcome is found in patients receiving OK-432 [7, 15, 24, 26, 36, 40]. We have performed a phase I study in 41 patients with advanced malignant disease receiving different doses of OK-432 by different routes to evaluate side effects and possible clinical benefits in patients, and to test immune modulating properties of OK-432 [24,25].

3.4.2.1. Single route
One single dose of 1 KE was given to 15 individual patients (12 malignant melanoma, 2 gastrointestinal and 1 breast carcinoma). In some of these patients NK-cell activity was monitored for at least 1 week and found significantly changed (see above). Side effects were mainly associated with the iv route [25].

3.4.2.2. Frequent application
Single route (14 patients) malignant melanoma stage III (Table 3.V). Six patients received OK-432 iv, 3 patients im, 4 patients it, and 1 patient id. A total dose of 24 KE was given iv to one individual patient. Two out of these six patients showed a transient tumor response. (Table 3.V). One of three patients, receiving OK-432 im (total dose 20 KE in several intervals) was maintained disease free for 18 months, in another patient the disease was stabilized for 4 months, one patient did not respond. Intratumoral injection of OK-432 led to one complete remission and to stabilization in two patients out of four.

⸴ One patient who had repeatedly developed lymph node metastases, despite intensive chemotherapy and/or radical surgery, received OK-432 intradermally. She was given weekly injections of 1–2 KE and after 1 month a complete remission of lymph node metastases was achieved. A pulmonary lesion present at the time of the therapy did not change during the further therapy course with OK-432 given for 3 months. In this patient, therapy is still continued.

Table 3.V.

Phase I study with OK-432. Frequent application in malignant melanoma (stage III)

Patient		OK-432 Dose		Response	
		Single	Total		
	iv Route				
1		1–3 KE	24 KE	PD	–
2		1 KE	16 KE	NC	3 MO
3		1 KE	7 KE	PR	3 MO
4		1–2 KE	7 KE	PD	–
5		1 KE	6 KE	PD	–
6		1 KE	3 KE	PD	–
	im Route				
7		1 KE	20 KE	NED	18 MO
8		1 KE	20 KE	NC	4 MO
9		1 KE	7 KE	PD	–
	it Route				
10		1 KE	3 KE	CR	10 MO
11		1 KE	3 KE	PD	–
12		1 KE	10 KE	NC	3 MO
13		5 KE	3 KE	PD	–
	id Route				
14		1–2 KE	24 KE	NC	4 MO

3.4.2.3. Combined routes

12 patients received OK-432 therapy by different routes at the same time, i.e. local (intralesional or perilesional injection) together with systemic im or iv. Five patients with advanced prostatic cancer were treated by combination of it and iv routes, but the results of these investigations are not yet conclusive. Seven patients (3 melanoma, 2 breast, 1 ovarian cancer and 1 hypernephroma) were also treated with combined routes. Local therapy resulted in partial remission in four patients. Furthermore, systemic disease, i.e. lung and liver metastases, was kept stationary for at least 3 months in two patients with malignant melanoma (Table 3.VI.).

From these studies we can conclude that OK-432 therapy has some effect on clinical outcome even in advanced cases of malignant disease, leading to some objective tumor response. Whether this is due to immune modulating effects and, possibly, due to interferon induction has to be further investigated.

Table 3.VI.

Phase I study with OK-432. Combined therapy with OK-432: systemic and local application

Patient	Disease (stage)	OK-432 (KE)		Therapy response	
		Syst.	Local	Syst/local	
1	Melanoma (III, lung, cutan.)	76 im	10 id	*NC/PR*	4 MO
2	Melanoma (III, lnn., liver)	30 iv	25 it	*NC/PR*	3 MO
3	Breast (IV, cutan.)	12 im	1 it	PD	–
4	Melanoma (III, liver, brain)	10 iv	9 it	PD	–
5	Breast (IV, lnn.)	4 iv	5 it	*—/PR*	4 MO
6	Ovarian (IV, asc.)	3 iv	3 ip	*—/PR*	2 MO
7	Hypernephroma (IV, cutan.)	3 iv	10 it	PD	–

3.4.2.4. Side effects
Both single and repeated injection (im, iv, ip, it, id) were well tolerated by all patients without severe side effects. The iv route led to fever and nausea in all patients investigated, starting 2 h after injection and lasting for 6–12 h. The other routes were without symptoms.

3.4.3. Randomized trial for adjuvant therapy of gastric cancer

Studies in Japan have already demonstrated some benefit of combining immunotherapy, i.e. OK-432, with chemotherapy in patients with gastric cancer. Both prolongation of disease-free interval and survival time has been reported [26,30]. In 1978 we initiated a trial to evaluate this combination therapy for patients after radical surgery of gastric cancer. In this study patients were randomized to receive either no further therapy (group A), chemotherapy (group B) or immuno-chemotherapy (group C).

The rationale for the use of immunotherapy before chemotherapy is given by the following observations: (1) Suppression of immune reactivity even in early stages of the disease and correlation of these parameters with prognoses. (2) Possible beneficial effect of immunotherapy given before chemotherapy, i.e. correlation of the immune status with response rate to chemotherapy [21,22].

Chemotherapy consisted of a three-drug combination which has been found effective previously for inoperable gastrointestinal cancers [26] and by ourselves.

3.4.3.1. Treatment regimen
Group A receives no further treatment. Group B: The regimens applied consist of

Cytosin–Arabinoside (Ara C) on day 1 (100 mg), Mitomycin C on days 1–4 (1 mg) and 5 fluorouracil on days 1–4 (12 mg kg^{-1}); this cycle is repeated every 6 weeks. A total of 3 cycles is given to the individual patients (Fig. 3.10).

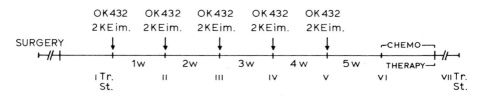

Fig. 3.10. Adjuvant therapy in gastric cancer. Outline of therapy regimen and timing.

Immunotherapy (group C) consists of one im injection of OK-432 weekly (2 KE per injection) for 5 weeks. One week after the last injection patients receive the same chemotherapy regimen as group B. Immunotherapy is given only in the initial therapy cycle. The time interval in groups B and C between surgery and chemotherapy is identical.

Follow up and clinical control is performed during the entire treatment period and then every 3 months for the first year, and is identical for all three groups. Relapse is confirmed by gastroscopy and X-ray examination. In case of early relapse therapy is discontinued.

Immune monitoring was performed to evaluate the influence of therapy; immune functions of patients, i.e. delayed cutaneous hypersensitivity reactions to recall antigens and to DNCB, was evaluated before and after each therapy cycle. Lymphocyte blastogenic response to mitogens was investigated before and during therapy and at the end of therapy. Serum lysozyme was used for monitoring macrophage secretory products and for correlating this with macrophage activity [6].

Furthermore, in some patients NK-cell activity was determined (as described above) during the initial immunotherapy and compared with patients receiving no therapy at this time in this study.

3.4.3.2. Clinical results

From 1978 to the end of 1980 59 patients have been included in the adjuvant therapy trial, and 52 are evaluable at present; 19 of them have been randomized to group A (no further therapy), 18 to group B, and 15 to group C. Relapse rates were 26% of patients (5/19) in group A, 27% (5/18) in group B, and 33% (5/15) in group C during the mean observation period of 55 weeks. Considering that the number of patients is too small and the observation period too short, these data cannot yet be regarded as conclusive. Due to randomization the number of patients in each group is not equally balanced. Nevertheless, all clinical parameters are comparable in each therapy group, i.e. surgical procedure (extended gastrectomy, gastrectomy or local resection), tumor extent and nodal status. None of the patients had distant metastases.

3.4.3.3. Immune monitoring

Most of the patients included in this study were also available for the evaluation of immune functions before and during therapy.

Delayed cutaneous hypersensitivity reactions to recall antigens did show differences within the therapy groups, when investigated before and after the first therapy cycle. Challenge tests performed with two concentrations of DNCB (100 µg and 50 µg) have revealed changes of the immune status of patients receiving immunotherapy with OK-432, as has already been found in the preliminary evaluation [25].

Table 3.VII.

Influence of therapy on DNCB reactivity

Therapy	DNCB 100 µg		DNCB 50 µg	
	Preth.	Follow up	Preth.	Follow up
A	9/10 90%	9/10 90%	4/10 40%	6/10 60%
		n.s.		n.s.
B	9/10 90%	6/10 60%	7/10 70%	5/10 50%
		n.s.		n.s.
C	6/13 46%	10/13 76%	4/13 30%	10/13 76%
		n.s.		$P<0.05$

Results expressed as number of patients with positive test/number of patients investigated.

In this evaluation, significant changes in skin test reactivity after the first therapy cycle were observed only in the group receiving the immunotherapy (Table 3.VII).

Before therapy 46% of the patients in group C (6/13) were found to react to DNCB 100 µg and 30% of them (4/13) to 50 µg DNCB. After the first therapy course including immuno- and, subsequently, chemotherapy, 76% of patients (10/13) were positive to the higher DNCB challenge dose and 76% (10/13) to the lower challenge dose ($P<$ 0,005, X^2 test).

An increase of DNCB reactivity has also been noted in the group receiving no further therapy, whereas the group with chemotherapy alone had a decrease. Both changes were without statistical significance (X^2 test).

Considering the conversion of DNCB reactivity after therapy in the different groups, it becomes evident that the highest numbers converting from DNCB negative to positive were found in the immuno-chemotherapy group (Table 3.VIII.). Furthermore a conversion from positive to negative was found in the two therapy groups but not in the OK-432 treated patients.

Table 3.VIII.

Conversion of DNCB reactivity during follow up

	Pos.[a] → Neg.		Neg.[b] → Pos.	
	100 µg	50 µg	100 µg	50 µg
A	1/9	2/4	1/1	4/6
B	3/9	2/7	0/1	0/3
C	0/6	0/4	4/7	6/9

[a] Number of conversions of patients initially positive.
[b] Number of conversions of patients initially negative.

From these results it can be concluded that OK-432 therapy has influenced immune reactivity of the patients when determined by DNCB reactivity.

Changes in lymphocyte blastogenic response and serum lysozyme – as a parameter for macrophage function [6] – have also been observed in patients receiving OK-432 therapy in this present trial and have been reported elsewhere [25].

NK-cell activity has already been found to be influenced by OK-432 in vivo and in vitro (see above).

In a preliminary study we investigated NK-cell activity against the K-562 cell line (for method see above) of two patients before and after OK-432 therapy and of two other patients included in these trials who were without therapy (i.e. arm A or B) for this time period (Table 3.IX).

All patients investigated were found to have low NK-cell activity after surgery. After OK-432 therapy reactions were found to be significantly enhanced ($P <$ 0.001; Student's t-test) when compared to those patients without therapy. This result suggests that OK-432 given sequentially for at least 5 weeks (im) is also

Table 3.IX.

Influence of OK-432 therapy on NK cell activity

Therapy	Cytotoxicity against K^{I}562 (%)		
	Before	Follow up	
None	11.3±5.2	14.6±7.2	
			P<0.001
OK-432	9.5±3.1	47.1±13.9	

E:T = 20:1. Results are expressed as % cytotoxicity (mean ± S.D. of two patients).

enhancing NK activity, similar to single intradermal and intravenous injections of 1 KE as observed in our Phase I study.

The immuno-chemotherapy regimen is well tolerated by all patients. There was no increase of toxicity by addition of immunotherapy. Nevertheless, the clinical results, regarding relapse rate, so far do not prove any advantage of one or the other therapy arm.

Results of immune monitoring give further evidence that OK-432 is a potent immune-modulating agent restoring DNCB reactivity, lymphocyte blastogenic response and possible increase of macrophage activity, (if lysozyme is a parameter allowing such a conclusion) and, furthermore, enhances natural killer cell activity.

3.5. DISCUSSION

The immune biology of cancer has now reached a state where several aspects of the immune mechanisms responsible for tumor cell elimination are becoming clearer [16]. Most progress has been obtained during recent years by the demonstration of natural cell-mediated immunity which is represented by natural killer cells [12,36] and macrophages [19]. Although the mechanisms of in vivo triggering of these effector cells are not clear, several animal studies and in vitro investigations with patients' peripheral blood cells, or cells derived from other body fluids or sources (i.e. ascites or pleural exudates or from draining lymph nodes), have given evidence that these natural defense mechanisms represent the first step in the elimination of tumor cells [11,12]. Although tumor-associated (specific?) antigens have been demonstrated in a variety of malignancies including melanoma [42], lung cancer [41], breast carcinoma [10], and further approaches can be expected from the use of monoclonal antibodies [42], the role of immunologic specific defense mechanisms against those antigens are not as clear as it was thought 10 years ago. At this time the first tests for demonstration of tumor-specific cellular and humoral immunity have been established. But, at present, there is no clearcut evidence that the demonstration of tumor-specific immune response in a cancer patient really reflects a prognostic factor or gives some information on the state of the disease. Nevertheless, several attempts have been made at inducing or potentiating immune mechanisms in the form of active specific immunotherapy by the use of intact tumor cells or tumor cell extracts. The other line of approach was to stimulate nonspecific defense mechanisms (active nonspecific immunotherapy) and, thus, increase and potentiate specific immunity. Although positive clinical effects have been achieved with both methods, no clear correlation with immune status (specific and nonspecific) has been obtained [2,22].

At present, most research is aimed at evaluating natural defense mechanisms in cancer patients and in screening for agents which are able to trigger these reactions. With the recent finding that interferon is able to enhance these natural killer mechanisms [11], several investigations have been performed to document clinical benefits from interferon, or to screen for agents which are inducing interferon and/or enhancing natural defense mechanisms. One approach might be the use of streptococcal preparation OK-432. We have demonstrated for the first time that OK-432 therapy is able to enhance natural killer cell activity in mice [43].

In the present investigation we have shown that different administration routes are also different in their efficacy of augmenting NK-cell killing of mouse spleen cells, i.e. the iv route seems to be the most effective. The therapeutic effect of OK-432 on the development of pulmonary metastases was also investigated. Again, iv application was found most effective in reducing the number of lung metastases in Lewis lung tumor-bearing mice.

Besides an immune modulating effect of OK-432 we have also observed that this preparation has a cytocidal effect on tumor cells in vitro, as demonstrated by time lapse cinematographic studies. Melanoma cells were inhibited in their mitotic activity upon incubation with OK-432. This confirms earlier studies in which OK-432 was found to inhibit the growth of a variety of tumor cells [30,33]. This direct antitumor effect might have some implication for local application of OK-432 [8]. We have already noticed some tumoricidal effect in patients with malignant melanoma, when OK-432 was applied intratumorally, i.e. into skin or lymph node metastases [24,25]. Besides the tumoricidal effect, the immune-modulating property also might have contributed to the tumor remissions observed.

Concerning the studies with human lymphocytes, we have demonstrated that OK-432, when incubated in vitro with peripheral blood mononuclear cells, is able to enhance killing against a natural killer-sensitive K-562 target cell line. This effect seems to be very rapid, as enhanced cytotoxicity was found to be present at 4 h, with a maximum after 20 h incubation. According to our investigations interferon seems not to mediate this effect, as supernatant recovered from lymphocyte cultures after OK-432 incubation did not augment the cytotoxicity of untreated effector cells.

The noted effect of enhancement of cytotoxicity was influenced by temperature, but not depressed by mitomycin treatment. Fractionation studies demonstrated, first, that macrophages are not important for enhancement of cytotoxicity and, second, that adherent and also non-adherent cells were rendered more cytotoxic after treatment with OK-432 in vitro. We found this effect comparable with that of interferon, although we feel that different mechanisms, according to these fractionation studies, are involved.

Recently we have also observed that OK-432 is able to reduce the activity of of suppressor cells to NK cells present in carcinomatous pleural effusions, which were found to be responsible for the lack of NK killing of lymphoid cells isolated from this fluid (Uchida, A., Micksche, M., in preparation).

Oshimi et al. [31] have recently also demonstrated that incubation of the lymphocytes of two normal donors with a variety of OK-432 doses in vitro enhanced the cytotoxicity against the K-562 cell line [31]. In patients with malignant melanoma and also stomach cancer we were able for the first time to demonstrate [25] that OK-432 therapy, given in a single or in several doses, is able to enhance NK-cell activity and that the iv route seems to be the most effective. Our results have been confirmed recently by Oshimi et al., who found that successive daily im and ip injection of OK-432 is able to enhance the cytotoxicity of cells obtained from peripheral blood and also of ascitic fluid, when compared with pretreatment values [31].

Induction of endogenous immune interferon by OK-432 therapy has already been reported by Matsubara in mouse systems [23]. Whether IFN is responsible for the observed increased NK killing after in vivo application of OK-432 has to be further confirmed. Concerning our phase I study it was demonstrated that the side effects (fever and nausea) of OK-432 therapy, appearing mainly when the preparation is given iv, are tolerable.

The clinical results of 27 evaluable patients (having received OK-432 for a longer time period) indicate some effects of this bacterial preparation, although it has been applied to patients in advanced stages of malignant disease. We observed a response at the tumor site such as an inhibition of disease progress for at least 3–4 months in five patients having received OK-432 by systemic routes. Local or intratumoral injection led to a partial remission in four patients, to a complete remission in one, and to stationary disease is another patient. Taken together, 11 out of 25 patients showed therapeutic responses after OK-432 application.

Immunotherapy of cancer with the *Streptococcus pyogenes* preparation OK-432 has been found effective in clinical studies performed in Japan [29]. In these investigations it has been proven that immunotherapy with OK-432 has some beneficial effect as an adjuvant therapy after radical or palliative resection of lung or gastric cancer [7,15,26,36,40]. Uchida et al. have recently demonstrated that OK-432 treatment of patients with adenocarcinoma of lung and stomach significantly prolonged survival times, in comparison to those of patients receiving chemotherapy alone [36]. Besides these clinical effects, increases of lymphocyte counts and lymphocyte blastogenic response, as well as normalization of the lymphocyte subpopulation's constitution, have been observed [36]. In another study the same authors found that suppressor cells, i.e. monocytes and nylon wool-nonadherent cells (which are supposed to be one of the causes of an impairment of cellular immune functions) are reduced after OK-432 therapy. In these patients, lymphocyte blastogenic response to mitogens, which was found depressed before therapy, reached normal level during treatment with OK-432 [37].

In our phase I study we have also found evidence that OK-432 therapy leads to immune restoration, since increase of lymphocyte blastogenic response and NK

52

killing has been observed [24,25].

The results of the adjuvant therapy trial should be considered preliminary because of the small number of patients included so far and the short follow-up period. Nevertheless, we found that OK-432 therapy significantly altered the DNCB reactivity of patients, suggesting that immunotherapy has at least a restoring effect on the immunosuppression related to malignant disease, previous surgery or subsequent chemotherapy.

From the investigations presented we conclude that the *S. pyogenes* preparation OK-432 is a potent immune modulator acting on NK cells, T-lymphocytes and, possibly, macrophages, thus activating the whole 'machinery' of cellular defense mechanisms which have been found important for tumor cell destruction, and besides this, OK-432 possesses direct cytocidal activity on tumor cells.

From the clinical data there is some evidence of the therapeutical efficacy of OK-432 even in advanced malignant disease. However, investigations in patients with better prognosis and lower tumor load are warranted for further documentation of the clinical usefulness of this *S. pyogenes* preparation.

The trial in patients with gastric cancer is in progress and further patient input and follow-up should give further evidence of the therapeutic usefulness of the OK-432 preparation.

REFERENCES

1 Aoki, T., Kvedar, J.P., Höllis, Jr, V.W. and Bushar, G.S. Brief communication: *Streptococcus pyogenes* preparation OK-432: Immunoprophylactic and immunotherapeutic effects on the incidence of spontaneous leukemia in AKR mice. J. Natl. Cancer Institute 56/3, 687, 1976.

2 Baldwin, R.W. and Pimm, M.V. Tumor immunotherapy – experimental evaluation and clinical prospects. in Immunodiagnosis and Immunotherapy of Malignant Tumours (H.D. Flad, Ch. Herfarth and M. Betzler Eds), p. 195, 1979, Springer Verlag; Heidelberg.

3 Chugai Pharmaceutical Co. Host defense stimulator: Antitumor *Str. pyogenes* preparation: Picibanil (OK-432) Compendium, 1977.

4 Coley, W.B. The treatment of malignant tumors by repeated inoculations of erycipelas with a report of original cases. Am. J. Med. Sci. 105, 487, 1893.

5 Colot, M., Müller, L., Yamagata, S. and Micksche, M. Immune modulation by BM 12 531 in vitro and in vivo. in Biology of Cancer Cells (K. Letnansky Ed.), p. 149, 1979, Kuler; Amsterdam.

6 Currie, G.A. Serum lysozyme as a marker of host resistance. II. Patients with malignant melanoma, hypernephroma or breast carcinoma. Brit. J. Cancer 33, 593, 1976.

7 Hattori, T., Niimoto, M., Yamagata, S., and Tohge, T. Clinical studies on streptococcal preparation (OK-432)* combined with mitomycin-C, 5-FU and cytosine arabinoside in advanced cancer patients. Jpn J. Surg. 5/3. 133, 1975.

8 Hattori, T., Niimoto, M., Yamagata, S., Tohge, T. and Terao, H. Experimental study on the effects of large-dose intratumoral OK-432 administration in mice. Gann 76, 105, 1976.

9 Havas, F.H.L., Donnelly, A.J. and Poreca, A.V. The cytotoxic effects of hemolytic streptococci on Ascites tumor cells. Cancer Res. 23, 700, 1963.

10 Herberman, R.B. Immunodiagnosis of human breast cancer. Cancer Detection and Prevention 1/2, 331, 1976.

11 Herberman, R.B., Djeu, J.Y., Ortaldo, J.R., Holden, H.T. West, W.H. and Bonnard, G.D. Role of interferon in augmentation of natural and antibody-dependent, cell-mediated cytotoxicity. Cancer Treatment Rep. 62/11, 1893, 1978.

12 Herberman, R.B., Djeu, J.Y., Kay, H.D., Ortaldo, J.R., Riccardi, C., Bonnard, G.D., Holden, H.T., Fagnani, R., Santori, A. and Puccetti, P. Natural killer cells: Characteristics and regulation of

activity. Immunol. Rev. 44, 43, 1979.

13 Ishii, Y., Yamaoka, H., Toh, K. and Kikuchi, K. Inhibition of tumor growth in vivo and in vitro by macrophages from rats treated with a streptococcal preparation OK-432. Gann 67, 115, 1976.

14 Johnson, A.G., Audibert, F. and Chedid, L. Synthetic immunoregulating molecules: A potential bridge between cytostatic chemotherapy and immunotherapy of cancer. Cancer Immunol. Immunother. 3, 219, 1978.

15 Kimura, I., Ohnishi, T., Yasuhara, S., Sugiyama, M., Urabe, Y., Fujii, M. and Machida, K. Immunochemotherapy in human cancer using the streptococcal agent OK-432. Cancer 37, 2201, 1976.

16 Klein, G. Immune and non-immune control of neoplastic development: Contrasting effects of host and tumor evolution. Cancer 45/10, 2486, 1980.

17 Kurata, T. and Micksche, M. Suppressed tumor growth and metastases by Vitamin A + BCG in Lewis lung tumor bearing mice. Oncology 34, 209, 1977.

18 Kurata, T. and Micksche, M. Correlation of immune response with clinical stage in Lewis lung tumor bearing mice. Oncology 35, 155, 1978.

19 Lemarbre, P., Hoidal, J., Vesella, R. and Rinehart, J. Human pulmonary macrophage tumor cell cytotoxicity. Blood 55/4, 612, 1980.

20 Mashiba, H., Gojobori, M. and Matsunaga, K. Antitumor effect of combined use of OK-432 and yeast cell wall with Mitomycin-C in mice. Gann 68, 703, 1977.

21 Mathé G. Immune status and cancer chemotherapy efficacy. Cancer Immunol. Immunother. 2, 81, 1977.

22 Mathé G. Systemic active immunotherapy is shifting from the Middle Ages to a Renaissance period. I. The multiplication of randomized trials showing significant effect of active immunotherapy on residual minimal disease. Cancer Immunol. Immunother. 5, 149, 1978.

23 Matsubara, S., Suzuki, F. and Ishida, N. Induction of immune interferon in mice treated with a bacterial immunopotentiator OK-432. Cancer Immunol. Immunother. 6, 41, 1979.

24 Micksche, M., Kokoschka, E.M., Sagaster, P. and Kofler, A. Klinische und immunologische Untersuchungen mit OK-432 (Streptococcus pyogenes) zur Immuntherapie bei Krebspatienten. Onkologie 1, 106, 1978.

25 Micksche, M., Kokoschka, E.M., Jakesz, R., Luger, Th., Rainer, R., Sagaster, P. and Uchida, A. Phase I study with Streptococcus preparation OK-432. in Immunotherapy of Cancer: Present Status of Trials in Man (W. Terry Ed.), 1982, Elsevier North-Holland; New York, in press.

26 Nakasato, H., Suchi, T. and Ota, K. Postoperative adjuvant immunochemotherapy for advanced carcinoma of the stomach with MFC and OK-432 (NSC-B116209). Cancer Treatment Rep., 1981.

27 Nauts, H., Fowler, G.A. and Bogatko, G.H. A review of the influence of bacterial infection and bacterial products (Coley's toxins) on malignant tumors in man. Acta Med. Scand. (Suppl.) 145, 1, 1953.

28 Okamoto, H., Shoin, S., Koshimura, S. and Shimizu, R. Studies on the anticancer and streptolysin S-forming abilities of hemolytic streptococci. A review. Jpn. J. Microbiol. 11, 323, 1967.

29 Okamoto, H., Shoin, S., and Koshimura, S. Streptolysin S-forming and antitumor activities of group A streptococci. in Bacterial Toxins and Call Membranes (J. Jeljaszewicz and T. Wadström Eds), 1978, p.259, Academic Press; London.

30 Ono, T., Kurata, S., Wakabayashi, K., Sugawara, Y., Saito, M. and Ogawa, H. Inhibitory effect of a streptococcal preparation (OK-432) on the nucleic acid synthesis in tumor cells in vitro. Gann 64, 59, 1973.

31 Oshimi, K., Wakasugi, H., Seki, H. and Kano, S. Streptococcal preparation OK-432 augments cytotoxic activity against an erythroleukemic cell line in humans. Cancer Immunol. Immunother. 9, 187, 1980.

32 Sakai, S., Ryoyama, K., Koshimura, S. and Migita, S.
Studies on the properties of a streptococcal preparation OK-432 as an immunopotentiator. Jpn. J. Exp. Med. 46, 123, 1976.

33 Sakurai, Y., Tsugagoshi, S., Satoh, H., Akiba, T., Suzuki, S. and Takagaki, Y. Tumor inhibiting

effect of a streptococcal preparation (NSC B 116209). Cancer Chemother. Rep. Part 1, 56, 9, 1972.

34 Stratton, M.L., Herz, J., Loeffler, R.A., McClurg, F.L., Reiter, A., Bernstein, P., Danley, D.L. and Benjamini, E. Antibody-dependent cell-mediated cytotoxicity in treated and non-treated cancer patients. Cancer 40, 1045, 1977.

35 Terry, W.D. and Windhorst, D. (Eds). Immunotherapy of Cancer: Present Status of Trials in Man. Prog. Cancer Res. and Therapy, Vol. 6, 1978, Raven Press; New York.

36 Uchida, A. and Hoshino, T. Clinical studies on cell-mediated immunity in patients with malignant disease. I. Effects of immunotherapy with OK-432 on lymphocyte subpopulation and phytomitogen responsiveness in vitro. Cancer 45, 476, 1980.

37 Uchida, A. and Hoshino, T. Reduction of suppressor cells in cancer patients treated with OK-432 immunotherapy. Internat. J. Cancer 26, 401, 1980.

38 Uchida, A. and Micksche, M. Natural killer cells in carcinomatous pleural effusions. Cancer Immunol. Immunother. 11, 131, 1981.

39 Uzi, S., Tanaka, J., Nomoto, K. and Torisu, M. Studies on the immune potentiating effects of a streptococcal preparation OK-432. I. Enhancement of T-cell-mediated immune response in mice. Clin. Exp. Immunol. 37, 98, 1979.

40 Watanabe, Y., Iwa, T. and Yamamoto, K. Clinical value of immunotherapy by streptococcal preparation, OK-432, as an adjuvant for resected lung cancer. 2nd World Lung Cancer Congress, Abstr. p 198, 1980.

41 Wolf, A., Micksche, M. and Bauer, H. An improved antigen marker of human lung carcinoma and its use in radioimmunoassay. Brit. J. Cancer 43, 267, 1981.

42 Woodbury, R.G., Brown, J.P., Yeh, M.Y., Hellström, I. and Hellström, K.E. Identification of a cell surface protein, p 97, in human melanomas and certain other neoplasms. Proc. Natl. Acad. Sci. USA 77/4. 2183, 1980.

43 Yamagata. S., Micksche, M., Al-Hashimi, M. and Vetterlein, M. Natural killer cell activity of mouse splenocytes against Lewis lung tumor cells. 5th Meeting EACR, Abstr. 40, p 44, 1979.

44 Yamagata, S., Koh, T., Oride, M. and Hattori, T. Antitumor effects of levamisole in combination with anaerobic *Corynebacterium*, OK-432 (streptococcal preparation), and chemotherapy in mice. Cancer Immunol. Immunother. 7, 217, 1980.

CHAPTER 4

Exploring the immunotherapeutic potential of two lipoidal amines

K.E. Jensen, J.F. Niblack, J.S. Wolff III, A.R. Kraska, I.G. Otterness, W.W. Hoffman and G.R. Hemsworth

Pfizer Central Research, Groton, Connecticut (USA)

4.1. INTRODUCTION

Since the days of Pasteur there have been research efforts to understand and manipulate responses of systems that engender immunity to infections. Vaccination to provide specific antigenic experience prior to encountering the disease agent has proven to be only one of several ways that resistance to disease can be increased significantly. Non-specific enhancement of host defenses can also be obtained; for example, administering materials that induce an interferon response is a powerful means of preventing viral infections. In addition, interferon is known now to modulate host defense systems in several ways including the activation of macrophages and augmentation of natural killer cells among T-lymphocyte populations.

Various kinds of microbial products have been found to activate macrophages; several of these substances are being widely studied and are the subjects of reviews elsewhere in this volume. Unfortunately, preparations of such natural materials frequently contain a spectrum of active moieties and therefore are difficult to standardize for quality control purposes. To circumvent these problems we have chosen to work with synthetic, low molecular weight compounds, and our group has discovered certain lipoidal amines that are inducers of interferon and/or activators of macrophages. Their potential uses as immunotherapeutants are being explored and some of the results obtained with two compounds will be described and reviewed here.

4.2. AN INDUCER OF INTERFERON, CP-20,961

This compound, with the structure diagrammed in Fig.4.1, has the chemical name *N,N*-dioctadecyl-*N'*,*N'*-bis(2-hydroxyethyl)propanediamine. It is the prototype of a large, structurally related series our research group began to characterize almost 10 years ago and which stemmed from efforts we initiated early in the 1960s to find substances capable of causing cells to make interferon. CP-20,961 was first reported 8 years ago as having antiviral activity and stimulating interferon production in mice [3]. Subsequent tests in human volunteers by intranasal instillation showed it to cause elaboration of interferon in nasal secretions and to reduce the severity of illnesses caused by interferon-sensitive rhinovirus strains [5]. Attempts to demonstrate interferon induction in vitro by this compound have not been successful; however, peritoneal macrophages recovered from mice dosed intraperitoneally with CP-20,961 a few hours earlier will secrete interferon. Summaries of these earlier research efforts with the compound and technical details of those experiments are reported elsewhere [3,5,6].

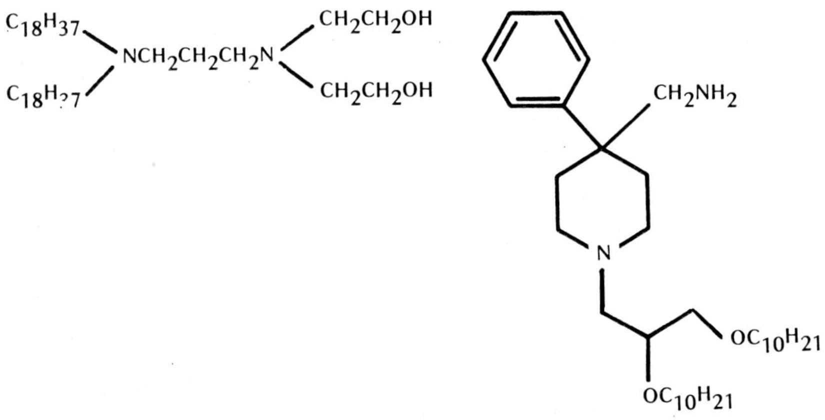

Fig. 4.1. Structures for CP-20,961, (*N,N*-dioctadecyl-*N'*-*N'*-bis[2-hydroxyethyl]-propanediamine); and CP-46,665, 4-Aminomethyl-1-(2,3-(di-*n*-decyloxy)-*n*-propyl)-4-phenylpiperidine.

4.3. THE VACCINE ADJUVANTING PROPERTIES OF CP-20,961

Noting that some interferon inducers can enhance immune responses, we examined the adjuvanting capacity of CP-20,961. This lipoidal diamine was found to be an excellent adjuvant for humoral and cell mediated immunity with many different kinds of antigens [6]. Comparisons with complete Freund's adjuvant (CFA) in the Lewis rat model of arthritis, and in guinea pigs injected with sheep erythrocytes or influenza vaccines have demonstrated that responses elicited with formulations of

CP-20,961 are equal or superior to those seen with CFA.

Studies by Anderson and Reynolds [1] with killed Venezuelan equine encephalitis virus vaccine revealed that CP-20,961 caused greater adjuvanting than did CFA of serum antibody titers and resistance to viral challenges. Their work also gave dramatic demonstrations that the mechanisms of action for this lipoidal amine and CFA are probably similar, in that they both cause increased lymphocytic traffic through regional lymph nodes where crescents of macrophages appear around germinal centers of the perifollicular mantel. Such macrophages are thought to be efficient processors of antigen for presentation to the T and B lymphocytic clones.

A most appealing feature of formulations containing CP-20,961 which differentiates it from CFA is that the subcutaneous or intramuscular injection site presents only a mild inflammatory cellular infiltration and this disappears in a few days [1,6]. There is no formation of granulomata or sterile abscesses such as commonly develop with use of CFA.

Recent extensions of information derived from other preliminary studies on the adjuvanting properties of this lipoidal amine have included finding significant enhancements of immune responses with a wide range of viral vaccines injected in mice, guinea pigs, swine and cattle. Experimental plasmoidal vaccines in cattle and monkeys also have been shown to be adjuvanted with CP-20,961 as well or better than that obtained with CFA or muramyl dipeptide preparations.

4.4. ANTITUMOR EFFICACY OF CP-20,961

Trials in rodents with tumor cell vaccines have demonstrated strong adjuvanting capacity with such antigens. Immunizations with EL4 cells mixed with CP-20,961 provided great increases of spleen cell cytotoxicity in vitro. In addition, injections of X-irradiated L-1210 cells to which this adjuvant had been added gave significantly increased resistance to challenge with live L-1210 cells [4,6]. Further explorations may be warranted using this adjuvant mixed with autologous tumor cells to examine the potential efficacy of treating tumor-bearing animals by specific enhancement of antigen-mediated reactions.

Non-specific host defense mechanisms that include macrophages alarmed by various substances are believed to have significant roles in resistance to or recovery from neoplasia. So it has become standard practice to determine whether immunotherapeutics have the capacity to activate macrophages. We have learned that cells contained in peritoneal washings from mice injected ip with the compound are activated to kill B-16 melanoma cells in tissue cultures. Approximately 1 mg kg^{-1} will induce that response in 48–72 h [6]. In contrast, the serum interferon induction and antiviral effectiveness is near maximal before 24 h and requires dosages in the 5–50 mg kg^{-1} range [3]. Conceivably this interferon is affecting a secondary (but with important augmenting actions) host defense system. CP-20,961 activates macrophages which not only kill tumor cells but also may secrete interferon. Interferon made by various kinds of cells including macrophages probably recruits killer cells from lymphocytic populations to help in the attack against cancer cells.

When tumor-bearing mice are treated with CP-20,961 improved survival rates can be seen and metastasis incidence is much reduced [4,6]. Table 4.I. lists data from experiments in CD-1 mice injected ip with 10^6 sarcoma 180J ascites cells. For those animals in which the compound was injected one day after tumor cell implantation, dosages as low as 8 mg kg^{-1} caused increased survival time. When treatment was not given for as long as 7 days, some effect could still be seen but only at higher dosages. Administration of drug prior to tumor cell implantation was also effective; the greatest increases in survival were obtained when the interval was 3–5 days before tumor cell injection. Evidently the antitumor efficacy is not dependent upon direct tumor cell killing; instead the observed lag period of 3 days suggests that such a time is required to recruit and activate macrophages and other antitumor cells.

Table 4.I.

Effects of CP-20,961 on the survival of mice with sarcoma 180

Dosage ip mg kg^{-1}		Treatment day	Mean days survival time	Increase % treated/control
0	Experiment A	–	20.3	–
8		+1	27.2	134
25			28.8(1[a])	142
75			33.7(3)	166
8		+4	19.3	–
25			26.2	129
75			23.5	116
		+7		
25			18.3	–
75			26.2	129
0	Experiment B	–	16.2	–
50		–1	23.8	147
		–3	31.3	193
		–5	28.0	173
		–7	21.8	134
		–9	17.8	110

[a] Number of animals, from groups of 6, that survived until test terminated on day 40.

The B-16 melanoma in C57 B1/6 mice can provide an excellent model of metastasis to the lung. For work reported here, tumor cell homogenates were implanted in a hind leg footpad and a tumor developed which was surgically removed on day 21 by amputation of the leg at the hip. If not further treated, these mice had a mean survival time of about 56 days. When killed on day 50 and the lungs examined macroscopically, we found in 35 control experiments using a total of 322 mice that 62% of the operated mice had more than five black melanotic lesions on their lungs (many had more than 50% of the lungs filled with tumor).

About 19% had 1–5 lesions per lung and 19% were lesion free. As shown in Table 4.II, if the operated mice were treated with doses of compound at 2.5 mg kg^{-1} or greater, there was significant inhibition of lung lesions. In these protocols the drug regimen was every fourth day beginning the day after surgery. Injections by either the intravenous or intramuscular route were effective.

Table 4.II.

Antimetastatic activity of CP-20,961 in mice with B-16 melanoma

Treatment	Dose (mg kg^{-1})	Regimen	Route	Mice with melanotic lesions (%)				
				N	>5/lung	1–5/lung	0	P values
Surgery + placebo	–	–	iv	322	52	19	19	–
Surgery + CP-20,961	0.6	q4d×4	iv	8	50	25	19	NS
	2.5	begin		8	25	38	38	<0.05
	10.0	day 22		8	38	12	50	<0.05
	40.0			8	12	25	83	<0.003
	0.6	q4d×4	im	8	75	12	12	NS
	2.5	begin		8	25	12	63	<0.005
	10.0	day 22		8	0	50	50	<0.002
	40.0			8	0	63	37	<0.005

Primary tumors were started by injection of tumor homogenates in the footpad of the left hind leg; removed by leg amputation at the hip on day 21. At autopsy on day 50 black lung lesions were counted.

4.5. COMPOUND FORMULATION AND ANIMAL TOXICOLOGY

The lipoidal nature of this substance makes it insoluble in water. Early formulations utilized Tween–glycerin mixtures and were fine particle suspensions, but the more recent preparations have been ethanol–Tween 80 solutions which are then mixed with a commercial soybean emulsion (Intralipid®, Cutter Laboratories, Fairfield, N.J.).

When formulated as Tween–glycerol suspensions, the acute LD$_{50}$ in mice intraperitoneally is >2000 mg kg^{-1} and intravenously is approximately 70 mg kg^{-1}. In Intralipid®, the acute iv LD$_{50}$ is 145 mg kg^{-1}, a 2-fold improvement. Oral absorption, to any substantial degree, has not been observed. Chronic toleration of the Tween–glycerol suspension was studied in dogs at 5 mg kg^{-1} iv daily for 28 days and no gross or histopathologic lesions were found in any organs; blood chemistry was unchanged [5].

4.6. CP-46,665, A VERY DIFFERENT LIPOIDAL AMINE

During a directed synthesis project to find new agents among lipoidal amines that would have immunomodulatory properties, compounds with several different structures were found that did not induce interferon but which had pronounced antitumor activities and would activate peritoneal macrophages [7]. One of them, coded CP-46,665, which was selected for further study was 4-aminomethyl-1-(2,3-(di-*n*-decyloxy)-*n*-propyl)-4-phenylpiperidine and has the structure shown in Fig.4.1. A commonality with CP-20,961 is their two long carbon chains (this one has 10 carbon atoms in each chain, while CP-20,961 has 18), and of course they both have amine groups. In contrast to the water insolubility of CP-20,961, water solutions of 50 mg ml^{-1} of CP-46,665 as a dihydrochloride salt are easily prepared. However, we found that iv administration of the compound to rodents and dogs in the lipid emulsion vehicle Intralipid®, was better tolerated and more effective than when given as a water solution.

From our point of view a major difference in the pharmacologic actions of the two compounds is that CP-46,665 does not induce interferon production in test animals. However, like CP-20,961, it is a macrophage activator. When the compound is injected intraperitoneally and peritoneal cells are collected 3 days later, significant cytotoxicity against B-16 target cells in vitro is observed. Single doses of 0.6 mg kg^{-1} were sufficient to cause the macrophage-like peritoneal cells to be cytolytic for the tumor cells. With L-1210 leukemia cells as targets in a thymidine uptake assay, the peritoneal macrophages were also seen to be highly active. Mice injected ip with only 0.3 mg kg^{-1} developed peritoneal exudate cells in 3 days, which produced 56–60% inhibition of L-1210 metabolism [7]. We conclude that CP-46,665 is an even more potent activator of macrophages than is CP-20,961. However, when stimulated with this compound the activated cells do not make interferon as do the peritoneal exudate cells collected from mice injected ip with CP-20,961 [6].

4.7. OTHER IMMUNOTHERAPEUTIC PROPERTIES

Mice bearing L-1210 leukemia lose their capacity to demonstrate a delayed hypersensitivity reaction to the contact-sensitizing agent oxazolone [2]. If they are treated ip with CP-46,665 (1.25 mg kg^{-1}) at 3 days after the L-1210 implant, a normal responsiveness to the sensitizing chemical is evident on the sixth day. Although the drug does not stop the leukemia and treated animals die at about the same time as controls, these results support the conclusion that CP-46,665 stimulates components of cell-mediated immunity which participate in this cutaneous reaction.

This compound has also been shown to adjuvant responses when mixed with vaccines. When influenza virus vaccines containing 5 mg of the compound in Intralipid® were injected intramuscularly in guinea pigs, hemagglutination-inhibiting antibody titers were greater than in the control vaccinated group and maintained at higher levels during the secondary response monitored at 65 and 100 days post-vaccination. When the compound was mixed with X-irradiated L-1210 cells a significant enhancement of immune response occurred as measured by increased life span following challenge with live L-1210 cells. Although the

Intralipid® vehicle control may have displayed some adjuvanting capacity (because it contains soybean oil and other lipids), significantly greater increments of immune enhancement were evident in vaccines containing the CP-46,665. We have concluded that both CP-20,961 and CP-46,665 are effective adjuvants in addition to their other immunotherapeutic actions.

Table 4.III.

Antimetastatic activity of CP-46,665 in mice with B-16 melanoma

Treatment	Dose (mg kg⁻¹)	Regimen	Route	Mice with melanotic lesions (%)				
				N	>5/lung	1–5/lung	0	P values
Surgery + placebo	–	–	iv	322	52	19	19	–
Surgery + CP-46,665	0.6	day 22 only	iv	16	19	50	31	<0.01
	2.5			16	25	31	44	<0.005
	10.0			16	38	25	37	<0.05
	0.6	q7d×3	iv	16	25	25	50	<0.005
	2.5	begin day 22		16	25	19	56	<0.005
	10.0			16	38	31	31	<0.1

Primary tumors were started by injection of tumor homogenates in the footpad of the left hind leg; removed by leg amputation at the hip on day 21. At autopsy on day 50 black lung lesions were counted.

4.8. ANTIMETASTIC DEMONSTRATIONS

As with CP-20,961 we have found this compound will also decrease lung metastatic lesions in the murine B-16 model where the primary tumor is removed by leg amputation. In mice injected intravenously with CP-46,665 prior to surgery only minor reductions in lesion incidence were obtained. But when treatment was started on the day after surgery most of the mice benefited and the number of animals that became disease and lesion free was more than double that found in control groups [7].

As shown in Table 4.III. weekly iv injections beginning the day after surgery provided very significant reductions in incidence of lung lesions with doses as low as 0.6 mg kg⁻¹. Preliminary experiments using cytoreductive drugs, like cyclophosphamide, have been tried in combination with this lipoidal amine and administered after surgery, also have given very encouraging results [7].

Another model of metastasis using the rat mammary adenocarcinoma 13762, has also been responsive to iv treatment with CP-46,665. Surgical removal of the primary tumor at 10 days after subcutaneous implantation results in visceral metastasis and death among untreated animals. When weekly injections were given, starting on the day of surgery, doses as small as 0.15 mg kg⁻¹ inhibited metastatic disease in many of the rats [7]. Trials with other models of metastasis are warranted.

4.9. RESPONSES OF RODENTS WITH SOLID TUMORS TO TREATMENT WITH CP-46,665

Testing of the compound against solid tumors without surgical intervention has yielded variable results [7]. Intralesional injections of mice bearing subcutaneous tumors of CaD_2 mammary adenocarcinoma or of B-16 melanoma retarded the growth rate of those lesions, but did not affect growth of tumors on the contralateral flank. Attempts to modify growth rates of these primary tumors by iv injections were unsuccessful. In contrast, rats bearing the Walker 256 carcinosarcoma implanted in the flank were responsive to treatments by iv injections of the drug. Doses as low as 0.2 mg kg^{-1} were seen to render almost half of the animals disease free at 100 days. Apparently these differences in response to treatment reflect significant variation among the model tumors in their sensitivities to immunotherapeutants. Notable also are observations suggesting variations among individuals within treatment groups in their capacity to benefit from the effects of compound administration.

4.10. TOXICITY AND TOLERATION DETERMINATIONS

In vitro tests have shown that CP-46,665 concentrations of 10^{-5}M or greater will cause lysis of B-16 melanoma and at 10^{-7}M the metabolism of spleen lymphocytes is inhibited. These observations cause questions to be raised concerning the possibility that the compound has some direct actions on tumor cells in vivo. The effects seen on splenic lymphocytes would be reason to predict that some severe damage to the spleen might become evident when the compound is administered chronically. Instead, only minor degrees of splenic hyperplasia have been observed in dogs and rats treated iv at 25 mg kg^{-1}; apparently this is another case where data from in vitro tissue culture experiments are not predictive for in vivo results. Mice and rats show an iv LD_{50} of 60–75 mg kg^{-1}; rats tolerated daily iv doses of 12.5 mg kg^{-1} for 14 days without evidence of toxicity. Dogs have received 25 mg kg^{-1} chronically (every 4 days for 3 months) with only minor alterations in hematological and blood chemistry profiles [7].

Toleration studies have also been conducted in clinical populations of dogs and cats with various kinds of spontaneous neoplasias. Dosages as high as 5 mg kg^{-1} were administered weekly for as long as 30 weeks. No adverse effects were found and partial curative responses were noted in a few cases with both species of animals (MacEwen, E.G., personal communication).

4.11. CURRENT DIRECTION OF RESEARCH

We have found that CP-20,961 and 46,665 are representatives of structural classes of lipoidal amines which have immunomodulatory properties such as the capacity to induce interferon, to activate macrophages, to inhibit neoplastic disease and to function as superior adjuvants for immune responses. We intend to study their immunotherapeutic potential in a wide spectrum of applications, including various forms of cancer and other conditions that could be favourably influenced by the pharmacological actions of these novel drugs.

REFERENCES

1 Anderson, A.O. and Reynolds, J.A. Adjuvant effects of the lipid amine CP-20,961. J. Reticuloendothel. Soc. 26, 667, 1979.
2 Hemsworth, G.R., Wolff, J.S. III, Kraska, A.R. and Jensen K.E. Delayed cutaneous hypersensitivity to oxazolone in mice with tumors. Cancer Res. 38, 907, 1978.
3 Hoffman, W.W., Korst, J.J., Niblack, J.F. and Cronin, T.H. N-N-Dioctadecyl-N',N'-bis(2-hydroxyethyl)propanediamine: Antiviral activity and interferon stimulation in mice. Antimicrob. Agents Chemother. 3, 498, 1973.
4 Kraska, A.R., Hemsworth, G.R., Hoffman, W.W. and Wolff, J.S. III. Antitumor activity of CP-20,961 and CP-28,888. Current Chemotherapy and Infectious Disease Proceedings of the 11th ICC and the 19th ICAAC. Vol. II, p. 1605. American Society for Microbiology, Washington, DC. 1980.
5 Niblack, J.F. Studies with low molecular weight inducers of interferon in man. Tex. Rep. Biol. Med 35, 528, 1977.
6 Niblack, J.F., Otterness, I.G., Hemsworth G.R., Wolff, J.S. III, Hoffman, W.W. and Kraska, A.R. CP-20,961: A structurally novel, synthetic adjuvant. J. Reticuloendothel. Soc. 26, 655, 1979.
7 Wolff, J.S. III, Hemsworth, G.R., Kraska, A.R., Hoffman, W.W., Figdor, S.K., Fisher, D.O., Jakowski, R.M., Niblack, J.F. and Jensen, K.E. CP-46,665-1: A novel lipoidal amine with antimetastatic and immunomodulatory properties. Cancer Immunol. Immunother. 12, in press, 1982.

CHAPTER 5

Klebsiella pneumoniae RNA as an immunomodulating and anti-tumor agent

B. Serrou[a], A. Rey[a], D. Cupissol[a], C. Estève[a], L. Dussourd'D'Hinterland[b], G. Normier[b] and A.M. Pinèle[b].

[a]Laboratoire d'Immunopharmacologie des Tumeurs INSERM U-236, ERA-CNRS NO.844, Centre Paul Lamarque, Montpellier (France); and [b]Centre d'Immunologie et de Biologie P. Fabre, Castres (France)

5.1. INTRODUCTION

Ribosomes are intracytoplasmic, inframicoscopic organelles which play a major role in protein synthesis [1]. They assure the transmission of the genetic information contained in the nucleus. This information passes into the cytoplasm as messenger RNA which is translated into polypeptide chains. Recent findings have generated interest in bacterial extracts as agents capable of stimulating immune response [6]. Studies of this type were prompted by the fact that whole attenuated bacteria such as mycobacteria [14] or *Corynebacterium parvum* [10] were found to elicit non-specific immunological stimulation and retard tumor growth. Among the extracts studied, those from ribosomes have drawn particular attention and have benefited from several years of research [21]. Some authors have suggested that RNA transmits specific immunological information regarding cytotoxicity vis-à-vis tumor cells [6]. This hypothesis has yet to receive final confirmation.

Non-specific stimulation of the immune system is, and has been, a source of encouraging anti-tumor effects in experimental immunotherapy, including that involving human trials [14]. Even without delving into more general pathological implications, these events suggesting the possibility of an agent which can stimulate the non-specific immune system would more than justify further investigation. The present paper concerns the evaluation of RNA ribosomal extracts from *Klebsiella pneumoniae*, both in vivo to study their anti-tumor activity and in vitro, focusing on selected individual immune functions. Phase I human trials involving immunodepressed patients with advanced tumor appear wholly justified based on the results reported herein and the low toxicity of ribosomal RNA extracts.

5.2. MATERIALS AND METHODS

5.2.1. Preparation and characterization of ribosomal RNA from K. pneumoniae (D.2000)

5.2.1.1. Culture conditions

K. pneumoniae biotype a were harvested from a fermentation flask following culture in medium containing 20 g beef extract, 20 g yeast extract, 20 g saccharose and 5 g sodium chloride per liter of medium at pH 7.

Cultures were incubated at 37°C and pH 7 at 25% oxygen saturation. Frothing was chemically inhibited. A growth curve was continuously recorded photometrically.

Culture time was 3h after which the cells were blocked in the exponential phase by rapid chilling to 10°C. Cells were then recovered by centrifuging, washed in physiological saline and reconcentrated by centrifugation. Cells are then stored frozen in sterile containers and monitored for bacterial contamination.

5.2.1.2. Ribosome isolation

The cell pellet was thawed as needed and resuspended in 0.01 M Tris–HCl buffer containing 0.01 M $MgCl_2$ and 0.15 M NaCl (pH 7.2; 0°C). The suspension was homogenized at low temperature in a microbead homogenizer, then centrifuged at $7\,500 \times g$ for 10 min, $30\,000 \times g$ for 45 min and $50\,000 \times g$ for 20 min, all at 0°C. The ribosomes reside in the clear supernatant which was placed in an ultracentrifuge at $140\,000 \times g$ for 150 min at 0°C. The crude ribosome pellet was resuspended in 0.01 M Tris–HCl at pH 7.2 containing 0.01 M $MgCl_2$ and left in contact with 0.25% sodium dodecyl sulfate (SDS) for 30 min at 20°C.

The washed ribosomes were recentrifuged at $140\,000 \times g$ for 150 min at 17°C. The ribosome pellet was resuspended in 0.1 M phosphate buffer at pH 6.0 and allowed to stand overnight at 4°C. On the following day this solution was centrifuged at $30\,000 \times g$ for 30 min and the ribosome-rich supernatant recovered for extraction of ribosomal RNA.

5.2.1.3. Extraction of ribosomal RNA

The ribosomal RNA was extracted in 80% phenol equilibrated with 0.1 M phosphate buffer at pH 6.0 containing 0.001 M sodium EDTA and 0.5% SDS. The first extraction employed 1 volume of phenol at 65°C for 10 min. The solution was chilled in an ice bath and the aqueous phase recuperated by centrifugation at $10\,000 \times g$ for 10 min at 0°C followed by a second extraction under the same conditions using a half volume of phenol. The final aqueous phase was extracted three times with 1 volume of ether to eliminate any residual phenol and bubbled to remove traces of ether.

The solution was adjusted to 0.1 M with NaCl and RNA precipitated in 2 volumes of ethanol over 4 h at −20°C.

The ribosomal RNA precipitate was resuspended in 0.05 M Tris–HCl buffer at pH 7.5, yielding a final concentration of 3–5 mg RNA per ml.

5.2.1.3. Purification of ribosomal RNA

To one volume of ribosomal RNA solution, 0.1 volume of 5% cetyltrimethylammonium bromide (CTAB) was slowly introduced applying constant agitation. The solution was incubated on ice for 5 min and the resulting RNA precipitate centrifuged at 10 000×g for 10 min at 4°C.

The pellet was then repeatedly washed with an excess of 70% ethanol containing 0.2 M sodium acetate at pH 7.0.

The washed precipitate was resuspended in 0.15 M NaCl, dialyzed against the same solution and sterilized by filtration through a 0.22 μm membrane.

5.2.1.4. Analytic methods

5.2.1.4.1. RNA determination RNA concentration was directly measured spectrophotometrically by scanning the 200–320 nm range. The 258 nm reading is directly proportional to the RNA concentration: 0.02 absorbance (A) units corresponds to 1 μg RNA per ml. The ratio $A280/258$ nm reflects the quality of the RNA preparation.

5.2.1.4.2. Qualitative analysis of RNA Several methods were employed to assure a quality RNA preparation, e.g. sucrose gradient ultracentrifugation followed by characterization of 16 S and 23 S RNA. A second technique employed high performance liquid chromatography (HPLC) of a perchloric acid hydrolysate which permitted evaluation of A, U, G and C bases and detection of thymine.

RNA preparations were also evaluated measuring change in the hyperchromic effect following treatment with pancreatic ribonuclease.

5.2.1.4.3. DNA determinations In addition to thymine detection by HPLC, DNA was measured using the Burton reaction [3].

5.2.4.4.4. Protein determinations Protein was measured by the Lowry et al. method [12] as well as amino acid determinations using the ninhydrin method of Moore and Stein [15] after 6 M HCl hydrolysis at 110°C.

5.2.4.4.5. Neutral hexoses determinations This was carried out using the anthrone reaction of Scott [20].

5.2.4.4.6. Hexosamine determination The test employed was the *para*-dimethylaminobenzaldehyde method of Elson Morgan [9].

5.2.4.4.7. Lipopolysaccharide determination (LPS) This was carried out using the carbocyanin color reaction of Jandra (11) and the Limulus test.

5.2.2. Tumor system

Experiments were carried out on C57 B1/6 mice, 6–8 weeks old which were allowed food and water ad libitum. The mice presented with either methylcholanthrene-induced tumor (which has been developed and characterized in the authors laboratory) [17] or Lewis tumor. For both tumors, 2×10^6 cells were implanted subcutaneously into the left hind limb. Death followed at an average 28 days later accompanied by multiple lung metastases which arise between the 7th and the 11th day.

The effects of RNA on tumor were evaluated according to the following criteria: tumor weight and volume (measured on days 7, 14, 21 and 28 post-implantation), the number of lung metastases (for Lewis tumor) and survival time. Thymus and spleen weights were also recorded.

In addition, we evaluated the effect of ribosomal RNA on the induction phase of methylcholanthrene tumor. 5 mg of methylcholanthrene on a disk was subcutaneously injected.

Results were judged by comparison with a control group in order to establish the time at which tumor appeared and survival.

5.2.3. In vitro evaluation of human lymphocytes

The same ribosomal RNA extract was evaluated for its effect on auto-rosette forming cells (ARFC) and NK activity.

5.2.3.1. Assay for auto-rosette forming cells (ARFC)

The technique employed was that of Caraux et al [2–4]. Briefly, 0.20 ml of lymphocyte suspension (10^7 cells per ml) was preincubated for 30 min at 4°C with 0.05 ml autologous serum. 0.05 ml autologous erythrocytes (auto-RBC) (3×10^8 per ml) were added to the lymphocyte-serum suspension which was centrifuged at $200 \times g$ for 5 min and incubated overnight at $+4$°C. ARFC were counted the following day using a hemocytometer. An auto-rosette was defined as a lymphocyte binding three or more auto-RBCS.

The effect of ribosomal RNA was evaluated following incubation of RNA with test lymphocytes prior to addition of auto-RBCS. The concentrations of RNA tested were 10^{-3}, 10^{-2} and 10^{-1} mg per ml per 10^7 lymphocytes.

5.2.3.2. NK activity

This parameter was evaluated using cells from the K562 line [13] originating from chronic myeloid leukemia. The cells were tagged with ^{51}Cr by incubation at 37°C for 2 h. The cells were then washed and constituted the target cells for the NK assay. 10×10^3 target cells were incubated at 37°C for 18 h in contact with test lymphocytes. The effector-target (E/T) cell ratios employed were 6/1, 12/1, 25/1 and 50/1.

Results were expressed as the percentage of cytotoxicity calculated as follows: $NK\ (\%) = (R—RS)/(RM—RS) \times 100$. R was the radioactivity in the supernatant at the end of incubation, RS was the radioactivity of supernatant to which no lymphocytes were added (spontaneous cpm release); RM was the radioactivity observed following complete lysis by hydrochloric acid (total cpm).

The effect of ribosomal RNA was measured by incubating test lymphocytes with RNA for 1 h at 37°C prior to addition of target cells. RNA concentrations employed were the same as those for the ARFC assay.

5.3. RESULTS

5.3.1. Purification of ribosomal RNA

The results of the above-mentioned analysis were as follows.

RNA content was equal to or greater than 97% pure, demonstrating the characteristic 16 S and 23 S peaks following sucrose gradient ultracentrifugation.

Base analysis characterization of A,U,G,C and trace amounts of thymine indicated DNA contamination to be 0.1%, which was confirmed by the diphenylamine reaction.

Protein contamination was less than 0.25%; hexosamines less than 0.2%.

The carbocyanin test for LPS was negative and less than 0.001 by the Limulus test.

Table 5.I.

Methylcholanthren-induced tumor effect of *Klebsiella pneumoniae* on tumor-induction time

Groups	Positivity/time (days)	Survival/time (days)
Control		31 ± 1.31
Bacterial ribosomes (μg)		
250	+ 7	31.38 ± 1.92
500	+ 9	35.67 ± 1.97
750	+ 11	36.71 ± 1.38
Bacterial ribosomes + cell wall (μg)		
250	+ 2	30.33 ± 1.41
500	+ 1	31.33 ± 1
750	+ 3	31.55 ± 1.37
Ribosomal RNA (μg)		
200	+ 22	43.33 ± 3.27
300	+ 14	38.6 ± 3.65
500	+ 19	45.8 ± 0.84
Ribosomal RNA + cell wall (μg)		
250	+ 14	37.17 ± 5.04
300	+ 12	41.17 ± 0.75
500	+ 16	43 ± 0.89
Cell wall (μg)		
100	+ 3	36.55 ± 1.21
200	+ 4	37.14 ± 2.12
300	+ 5	37.6 ± 1.26

Table 5.II.

Effect of *Klebsiella pneumoniae* (KP) on methylcholanthren-induced tumors

Extract (µg)	Positivity (days)	P value
Bacterial ribosomes		
250	125 ± 3	<0.001
500	127 ± 3.2	<0.001
750	129 ± 4.5	<0.001
Bacterial ribosomes + cell wall		
250	120 ± 3	0.008
500	119 ± 4.5	0.46
750	121 ± 4	0.03
Ribosomal RNA		
200	140 ± 1.5	<0.001
300	132 ± 2.5	<0.001
500	137 ± 0.5	<0.001
Ribosomal RNA + cell wall		
200	132 ± 2	<0.001
300	130 ± 1.3	<0.001
500	134 ± 2	<0.001
Cell wall		
100	121 ± 4.8	<0.001
200	122 ± 2	<0.001
300	123 ± 2.5	<0.001
Control (no treatment)	118 ± 4	

5.3.2. Tumor system

5.3.2.1. The effect of ribosomal RNA extract from K. pneumoniae on the induction of a methylcholanthrene tumor

Methylcholanthrene tumor appeared on day 118 ± 4 after subcutaneous methylcholanthrene implantation in non-treated animals. Intra-peritoneal injection of bacterial ribosomes (with and without cell walls) or cell walls alone caused only a minimal but significant delay in the onset of tumor. The most significant results were obtained after injection of ribosomal RNA alone. Addition of cell walls did not improve upon these results. The effect was dose dependent since the results were essentially the same whether 200, 300 or 500 µg were injected. These results were paralleled by increased survival times, measured from the time the tumor became experimentally evident. Increased survival was also most significant for ribosomal RNA alone and independent of the dose employed. (See Tables 5.I. and 5.II.)

5.3.2.2. The effect on tumor growth in both tumor systems

The most significantly increased survival was noted for animals receiving ribosomal RNA. Addition of cell walls had no accrued benefit. A very significant increase in survival time was observed compared to control groups, the effect being independent of the dose. The results for Lewis tumor were identical, significant results only being observed for ribosomal RNA and were independent of the dose administered. It should be noted that results were always inferior whenever cell walls were added to RNA injections. There was also significantly decreased tumor weight, volume and number of metastases, as recorded on days 7, 14, 21 and 28 following tumor implantation, for the group receiving ribosomal RNA as compared to the other groups. (See Tables 5.III. and 5.IV.)

Table 5.III.

Effect of *Klebsiella pneumoniae* (KP) on methylcholanthren-induced tumors

Extract (μg)	Survival time (days)	P value
Bacterial ribosomes		
250	31.38 ± 1.92	0.51
500	35.67 ± 1.97	0.001
750	36.69 ± 1.38	0.001
Bacterial ribosomes + cell wall		
250	30.33 ± 1.41	0.4
500	31.33 ± 1	0.64
750	31.55 ± 1.37	0.75
Ribosomal RNA		
200	43.33 ± 3.27	0.001
300	38.6 ± 3.65	0.001
500	45.8 ± 0.84	0.001
Ribosomal RNA + cell wall		
200	37.17 ± 5.84	0.001
300	41.17 ± 5.04	0.001
500	43 ± 0.89	0.001
Cell wall		
100	36.55 ± 1.21	0.001
200	37.14 ± 2.12	0.001
300	37.6 ± 1.26	0.001
Control (no treatment)	31 ± 1.31	

Bone marrow cells or splenocytes from normal or tumor-bearing syngeneic mice did not affect tumor growth, number of metastases or survival following preincubation with different *K. pneumoniae* extracts and injected iv into tumor animals either on the same day as tumor implantation or 10 days after.

Table 5.IV.

Effects of *Klebsiella pneumoniae* (KP) on survival time (Lewis tumor)

Groups[a]	Days (µg)	Mean	± SD	P value
Control		28.33	± 2.35	
Bacterial ribosomes	250	29	± 1.05	0.58
	500	29.3	± 1.42	0.38
	750	29.5	± 1.78	0.22
Bacterial ribosomes + cell wall of KP	250	28.2	± 0.79	0.87
	500	28.6	± 0.70	0.73
	750	28	± 1.15	0.69
Ribosomal RNA	200	33	± 2.54	<0.001
	300	31.7	± 2.98	<0.01
	500	33.9	± 2.85	<0.001
Ribosomal RNA + cell wall of KP	200	29	± 1.76	0.48
	300	30.1	± 1.85	0.08
	500	30.2	± 2.15	0.08
Cell wall of KP	100	29.5	± 1.9	0.24
	200	28.9	± 2.13	0.68
	300	29.7	± 1.49	0.30

[a] Number of mice per group = 10.

In contrast (Table 5.V) thymocytes obtained from normal mice significantly prolonged survival of animals with methylcholanthrene or Lewis tumors. This effect was not enhanced following preincubation with ribosomal RNA. Thymocytes from syngeneic animals with the same tumor even more significantly prolonged survival of animals with the same tumor after iv injection either on the day of tumor implantation or 10 days afterward. If the same thymocytes were preincubated for 30 min in 20 or 50 µg ribosomal RNA per ml per 30×10^6 cells, survival was even more prolonged, resulting in four complete cures for the Lewis tumor group and two for methylcholanthrene tumor. There was no effect whatsoever when thymocytes from tumor animals were incubated with other ribosomal extracts.

One should note that a less significantly reduced thymus weight was observed for animals receiving ribosomal RNA, particularly as measured on the 21st and 28th day following implantation. This was concomitant with negligible variations for spleen weight compared to the other groups.

5.3.3. *In vitro effect on human lymphocytes*

Ribosomal RNA had no effect on ARFC in normal subjects, but caused a very significant increase in subjects with low ARFC levels where values as low as 9% can

Table 5.V.

Effects of KP RNA pre-incubated thymocytes on survival (days) of tumor-bearing mice (TBM)

Groups	Lewis tumor	Methylcholanthren tumor
Control medium	30.67 ± 0.52	37 ± 0.89
RNA 4 μg iv	36.83 ± 0.98	39.17 ± 1.17
RNA 10 μg iv	41 ± 0.89	40.17 ± 1.47
Normal thymocytes	45.17 ± 1.94	44.33 ± 0.82
RNA 20 μg pre-incubated normal thymocytes	44.17 ± 1.17	42.67 ± 0.92
RNA 50 μg pre-incubated normal thymocytes	46.83 ± 0.98	42.95 ± 0.80
Thymocytes from TBM	58.83 ± 0.98	45.33 ± 1.03
RNA 20 μg pre-incubated TBM thymocytes	69.2 ± 1.1	68.9 ± 1.1
RNA 50 μg pre-incubated TBM thymocytes	70 ± 1.32 (4 complete remissions)	75 ± 0.8 (2 complete remissions)

30×10^6 thymocytes were injected iv on the day and 10 days after tumor implantation. Incubation time, 30 min, 250 and 50 μg per ml per 30×10^6 cells; 10 mice per group.

rise to 24%. These were immunodepressed patients with advanced solid tumor. If one looks at the number of rosettes which form after 1 h (early ARFC) and those which occur after overnight incubation (late ARFC), a negligible effect can be attributed to early ARFC compared with a very significant effect on late ARFC. Early and late ARFC evaluate two different lymphocyte subpopulations, the early rosettes probably involving immature T cells, the other expressing Fc receptor for IgM [13,18].

Although isoprinosine, bestatine and interferon can significantly augment NK activity, no such increase can be attributed to *K. pneumoniae*. In fact, there was a very significant decrease wherein an initial value of 36% fell as low as 12%.

5.4. DISCUSSION

The present results clearly demonstrate that *K. pneumoniae* extracts can modulate host-tumor reactions and retard tumor growth. The most efficacious of these extracts appears to be ribosomal RNA. Methylcholanthrene induced tumor developed at a slower rate in response to ribosomal RNA, thereby leading to increased survival as measured from the time the tumor appeared. Animals with directly implanted methylcholanthrene or Lewis tumors present decreased tumor growth and increased survival time following intraperitoneal or intravenous injection of *K. pneumoniae* extracts, particularly ribosomal RNA.

The most striking results were observed following incubation of thymocytes from syngeneic tumor animals. We were surprised that no effect was observed for spleen or bone marrow cells from normal or tumor animals, since incubation in thymosin had previously been observed to exert a very definite influence [5]. An equally surprising result was that normal thymocytes as well as those from syngeneic animals with tumor, very significantly prolonged survival in animals with the same tumor. Moreover, preincubation of thymocytes from tumor animals in ribosomal RNA not only reinforced the previously observed effect but resulted in cases of complete cures for a tumor as difficult to treat as Lewis tumor. We offer no particular explanation for this kind of result, especially since up to now, thymocytes were more associated with enhanced tumor growth [20,16]. This could be related to the point in time at which thymocytes were obtained relative to tumor implantation. This possibility is presently being explored.

The effect brought about by thymocytes would lead one to believe that ribosomal RNA may exert its effect(s) on the T lymphocyte, although the exact thymocyte subpopulation involved has yet to be established. This point is also presently under investigation. The T lymphocyte effect is confirmed by in vitro results on ARFC. Ribosomal RNA very significantly augments ARFC levels, particularly the low levels observed for the immunodepressed patient with advanced tumor. This effect is particularly clear for late ARFC which correspond to a subpopulation with Fc receptor for IgM and which may be either the entire T lymphocyte population or helper cells [18]. Ribosomal RNA does not seem to augment in vitro NK function in the cancer patient, and may even cause it to decrease, although the significance of such a phenomenon is not clear if we take into account the suggested regulatory role of NK cells. The absence of enhanced NK activity was foreshadowed by the results of preincubation of ribosomal RNA with bone marrow cells resulting in no change in tumor growth.

Overall, these results suggest that ribosomal RNA from *K. pneumoniae* possesses anti-tumor properties although the mechanism remains unknown. This activity is observed following peritoneal or intravenous injection as well as introduction of preincubated thymocytes from syngeneic tumor animals. The point of impact seems to be a subpopulation of T lymphocytes since thymocytes from tumor-bearing animals present increased anti-tumor activity subsequent to injection with ribosomal RNA. Moreover this RNA very significantly increases the number of ARFC. These results confirm the general properties already observed for this type of extract with its efficacy as noted in other non-tumor models [7,8].

Taken as a whole, these results, and the minimal toxicity reported to date for this extract, warrant further investigation of its mechanism of action. In addition, initiation of in vivo human phase I trials to evaluate side-effects should be started and the in vivo point of impact that produces the immune response should be researched.

REFERENCES

1   Bosch, L. The mechanism of protein synthesis and its regulation. in Frontiers of Biology Vol. 27 (Neuberger, A. and Tatum, E.L. Eds), 1972, North-Holland; Amsterdam.

2   Boyum, A. Separation of leukocytes from blood and bone marrow. Scand. J. Clin. Lab. Invest. 21, 97, 1968.

3   Burton, J. DNA measurement with diphenylamine. Biochem. J. 62, 315, 1956.

4   Caraux, J., Thierry, C., Estève, C., Flores, G., Lodise, R. and Serrou, B. Human autologous rosettes. I. Mechanism of binding of autologous erythrocytes by T cells. Cell. Immunol. 45, 36, 1979.

5   Cupissol, D., Rey, A., Goldstein, A.L. and Serrou, B. Thymosin treated bone marrow cells retards growth in mice. 1981, submitted for publication.

6   Deloince, R., Beaudry, Y., Robert, D., Barjow, P., La Pivert, P. and Fontanges, R. Effet d'un mélange de ribosomes bactériens et d'une fraction membranaire de Klebsiella pneumoniae sur le développement d'un cancer épithélial greffé chez le rat. C.R. Soc. Biol. 171, 818, 1977.

7   De Vries, J.E., Mendelsohn, J. and Bont, W.S. The role of target cells, monocytes, and Fc receptor bearing lymphocytes in human spontaneous cell-mediated cytotoxicity and antibody dependent cellular cytotoxicity. J. Immunol. 125, 396, 1980.

8   Dussourd D'Hinterland, L., Pinèle, A.M. and Rey, G. Les vaccins ribosomaux : étude immunologique. Rev. Franc. Allergol. 17, 21, 1977.

9   Elson, L. and Morgan, W.T.J. A colorimetric method for the determination of glucosamine-N-chondrosamine. Biochem. J. 27, 1824, 1933.

10 Halpern, B. and Israel, L. Study of the action of an immunostimulin associated with anaerobic coryne bacteria in human experiental neoplasms. C.R. Acad. Sci. 272, 2186, 1971.

11 Jandra, J. and Work, E. A colorimetric estimation of lipopolysaccharides. FEBS Lett. 16, 343, 1971.

12 Lowry, O.M., Rosebrough, N.J., Farr, A.L. and Randall, R.J. Protein measurement with the folin phenol reagent. J. Biol. Chem. 193, 265, 1951.

13 Lozzio, C.B. and Lozzio, B.B. Cytotoxicity of a factor isolated from human spleen. J. Natl. Cancer Inst. 50, 535, 1973.

14 Mathe, G. Active immunotherapy of cancer: its immunoprophylaxis and immunorestoration. 1976, Springer-Verlag; New York.

15 Moore, S. and Stein, W.H. Modified ninhydrin reagent for the photometric determination of amino-acid and related compounds. J. Biol. Chem. 211, 907, 1954.

16 Reinisch, C.L., Andrew, S.L. and Schlossman, S.F. Suppressor cell regulation of immune response to tumors: abrogation by adult thymectomy. Proc. Natl. Acad. Sci. USA 74, 2989, 1977.

17 Reme, T., Gauci, L. and Serrou, B. Antigénicité des tumeurs chimio-induites chez la souris. II. Nature et spécificité de la réponse immune secondaire in vitro en culture mixte leucocytes-cellules tumorales. Ann. Immunol. Inst. Pasteur 1296, 766, 1978.

18 Rey, A., Rucheton, M., Caraux, J., Estève, C., Thierry, C. and Serrou, B. Autologous rosette forming cells: functional evaluation. 1981. Submitted.

19 Scott, T.A. and Melvin, E.H. Hexose determination with anthrone reagent. Anal. Chem. 25, 1956, 1953.

20 Umiel, T. and Trainin, N. Immunological enhancement of tumor growth by syngeneic thymus-derived lymphocytes. Transplantation 18, 244, 1974.

21 Youmans, G.P. and Youmans, A.S. Implications of immunization against infection diseases with ribosomal and RNA vaccines. in The Immune System and Infection Diseases. (4th International Convoc. Immunology, Buffalo, N.Y., 1974) p. 453, 1975, Karger; Basel.

CHAPTER 6

Bay i 7433, a non-ionic copolymer with anti-tumor activity

H.D. Schlumberger

Institute of Immunology and Oncology, Bayer AG, Wuppertal (FRG)

6.1. CHEMICAL AND PHYSICO-CHEMICAL PROPERTIES OF BAY i 7433

Bay i 7433 is a highly water-soluble, non-ionic copolymer that is obtained by the copolymerization of 30% (w/w) 1,3-bis(methylaminocarboxy)-2-methylene propane and 70% (w/w) N-vinylpyrrolidone. The schematic structure of this polymer is depicted in Fig. 6.1.

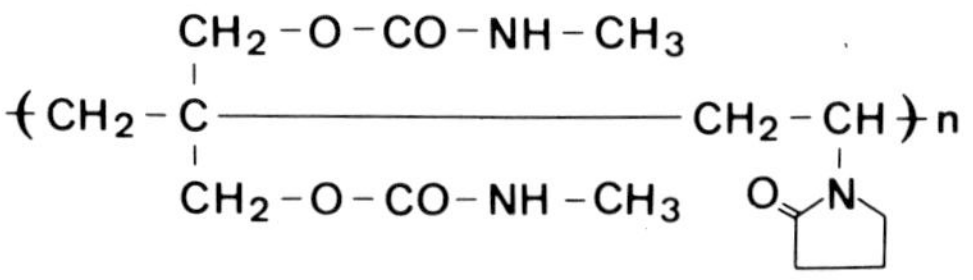

Fig. 6.1. Schematic structure of Bay i 7433.

The polymerization of the monomers results in a product with a narrow molecular weight distribution and a relatively uniform chemical composition. Gel chromatography on Fractogel^{TM} PVA 20 000 of Bay i 7433 in methanol yielded highly reproducible molecular weight distributions of different 10-kg batches (Fig. 6.2.). The average molecular weights of these preparations amount to 5800.

Preparative gel chromatography on Fractogel ^{TM} with methanol as the eluant and subfractionation of Bay i 7433 resulted in the cumulative molecular weight distribution as depicted in Fig. 6.3. The chemical composition with respect to the content of N-vinylpyrrolidone was determined by ^{13}C nuclear magnetic resonance of the different carbonyl residues. The content of N-vinylpyrrolidone increases

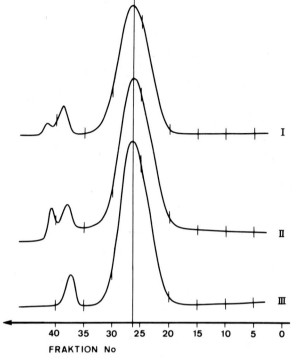

FRAKTION No

Fig. 6.2.   Gel chromatography (Fractogel[R] PVA 20 000 (Merck, Darmstadt, FRG)) of three 10-kg batches of Bay i 7433 in methanol. The effluent was monitored by differential refractometry. The small peaks at fractions 37–39 and 41 represent water and butyl acetate, respectively.

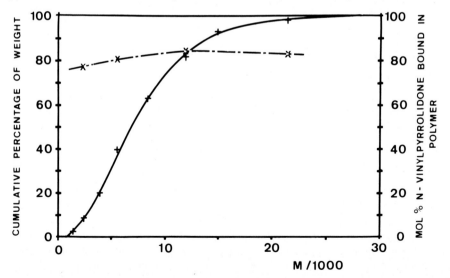

Fig. 6.3. Cumulative molecular weight distribution of Bay i 7433 after preparative fractionation by gel chromatography (same conditions as mentioned in Fig. 6.2.). The chemical composition with regard to the content of N-vinylpyrrolidone was determined by ^{13}C nuclear resonance.

slightly with increasing molecular weight which is to be expected from the preparation procedure of radical polymerization. The cumulative recoveries of nine fractions with different average molecular weights after preparative gel chromatography indicate a relatively narrow molecular weight distribution: 90% of the preparation has a molecular weight of more than 30 000. This molecular weight distribution would, thus, theoretically allow kidney passage.

6.2. INHIBITION OF TUMOR GROWTH

The anti-tumor activity of Bay i 7433 was investigated in the following experimental tumor systems.
1. Sarcoma 180 in outbred VRL mice (inoculation of 1.5×10^5 tumor cells).
2. Fibrosarcoma FIO 26 in C57 Bl/6 mice (inoculation of 2×10^5 tumor cells).
3. Carcinoma EO 771 in C57 Bl/6 mice (inoculation of 2×10^3 tumor cells).
4. Leukemia P 388 was propagated in B6 D2F$_1$ mice as a subcutaneous solid tumor after inoculation of $1-5 \times 10^4$ tumor cells.
5. Walker 1098 tumor in Wistar rats (inoculation of $2-4 \times 10^4$ tumor cells).

All tumors were inoculated subcutaneously unless otherwise stated. Inhibition of tumor growth was determined after administration of Bay i 7433 either prior to, or after tumor cell inoculation. The animals were sacrificed 21–25 days after tumor transplantation, and the tumors excised and weighed. In further experiments, the survival time of animals treated with Bay i 7433 was determined. Examples of these investigations are presented in the following pages.

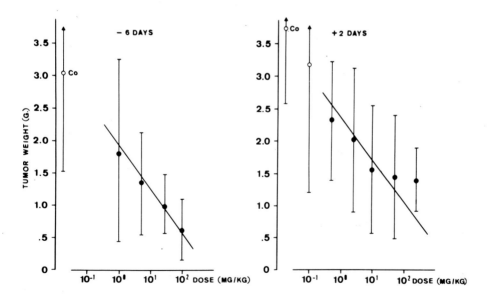

Fig. 6.4. Growth inhibition of carcinoma EO 771 after a single intramuscular administration of different doses of Bay i 7433 prior to (−6 days) or after (+2 days) inoculation of 2×10^3 tumor cells.

80

Carcinoma EO 771 is dose-dependently inhibited after a single intramuscular administration of the polymer given either prior to (prophylactic), or after (therapeutic) tumor cell inoculation (Fig.6.4.). When the compound is administered 6 days prior to tumor transplantation, tumor growth is significantly inhibited in a dose range of 1–1000 mg kg^{-1}. Maximal inhibition of 80% compared to the non-treated control animals is achieved at 100 mg kg^{-1}. The inhibitory dose range is similar when the polymer is given 2 days after tumor cell inoculation. The maximal inhibition of 60% is achieved with doses of 10 and 100 mg kg^{-1}.

Fibrosarcoma FIO 26 is similarly inhibited (Fig.6.5.). Prophylactic treatment 6 days before tumor transplantation results in a significant inhibition of the tumor growth in the applied dose range. The dose dependence in these experiments is certainly not strong and more complex relationships between dose and activity have to be assumed, e.g. a dose/time/activity relationship. The inhibitory dose range is 0.5–100 mg kg^{-1} after intramuscular injection of Bay i 7433. Significant and dose-dependent inhibition of tumor growth is achieved in the therapeutic regimen after a single injection of the polymer in a dose range of 1–100 mg kg^{-1}. The maximal tumor inhibition is 80–90% after prophylactic as well as therapeutic treatment.

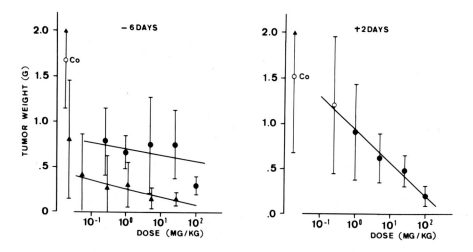

Fig. 6.5.   Growth inhibition of fibrosarcoma FIO 26 after a single intramuscular administration of different doses of Bay i 7433 prior to (−6 days), or after (+2 days) inoculation of 2×10^5 tumor cells.

In the next experiment (Fig. 6.6.), C57 Bl/6 mice were treated with 100 mg kg^{-1} Bay i 7433 three days prior to the inoculation with different numbers of carcinoma EO 771 cells. The animals were sacrificed 22 days after tumor cell inoculation, and tumor weights of controls and treated animals determined. Depending on the number of tumor cells inoculated, the tumor growth is significantly inhibited in the animals pre-treated with the compound. To achieve the tumor size of the non-treated controls, about 1000–2000 times more living tumor cells are necessary in the experimental group.

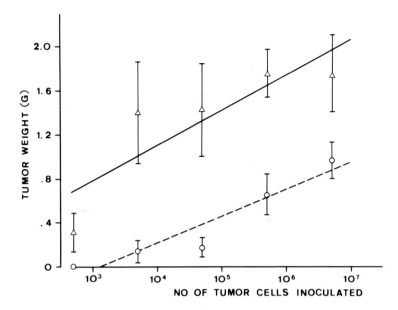

Fig. 6.6.   Inhibition of carcinoma EO 771 tumors by a single injection of 100 mg kg⁻¹Bay i 7433 three days before inoculation of different numbers of tumor cells. Controls received saline. The animals were killed 22 days after tumor cell inoculation. The tumors were excised and tumor weights recorded.

Intramuscular and intravenous application of the polymer were equally effective. These routes of administration were more effective and led to more consistent results than intraperitoneal or oral application. Oral application of the compound in a dose range of 50–500 mg kg^{-1} resulted in an inhibition of the tumor growth in the tumor systems investigated in an order of magnitude of 30–50%. Preliminary experiments suggested that local application at the site of excision of the primary tumors also resulted in an inhibition or retardation of tumor recurrences.

The inhibition of the growth of carcinoma EO 771 and sarcoma 180 after intramuscular administration of 50 mg kg^{-1} Bay i 7433 at different times in relation to tumor cell inoculation is shown in Fig. 6.7. In these experiments, the animals were treated with the polymer at different times prior to, or after tumor transplantation and were killed 20 days after tumor cell inoculation. The tumors were excised and weighed. The results are expressed in percent of the average tumor weights of the non-treated control groups. Anti-tumor activity is seen when the polymer is given 10 days prior to tumor transplantation. The activity decreases and the results become more inconsistent when the polymer is administered one or two days before tumor inoculation. After therapeutic treatment, the activity of Bay i 7433 decreases with increasing interval relative to tumor cell inoculation.

Multiple treatment with Bay i 7433 in various regimens proved to be no more effective than a single administration when evaluated by the tumor weight 21 – 25

82

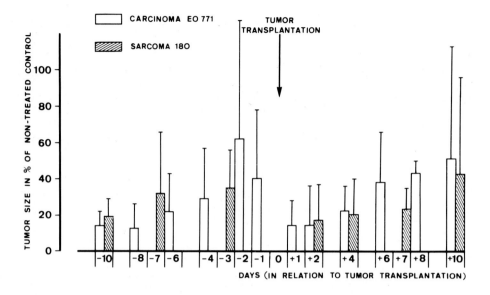

Fig. 6.7. Anti-tumor activity of Bay i 7433 after treatment at different times prior to, and after inoculation of carcinoma EO 771 or sarcoma 180 cells. The animals received a single injection of 50 mg kg^{-1} of the polymer at the times indicated. Controls received saline. The animals were killed 20 days after tumor transplantation. The results are expressed as the relative average tumor weights in comparison to the average tumor weights of the controls.

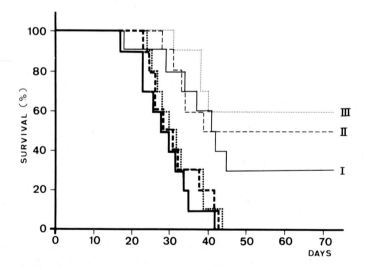

Fig. 6.8. Survival of carcinoma EO 771-bearing animals after one (I: 3 days prior to tumor transplantation (TT)), two (II: 3 days prior to, and 10 days after TT), and three (III: 3 days prior to, and 10 and 18 days after TT) intramuscular injections of 1 mg kg^{-1} Bay i 7433.

days after tumor cell inoculation. Treatment of animals with Bay i 7433 prior to or after tumor transplantation increases significantly the median survival time. However, in most experiments all treated animals die off and multiple treatment did not result in an improvement of the survival time. Only in a few experiments did some animals show a prolonged survival. An example of such an experiment is given in Fig. 6.8. A higher efficiency of multiple treatment, however, cannot be deduced from this experiment. Fig. 6.9. shows an experiment with 25 mg kg^{-1} Bay i 7433 given one day, 1 and 8 days and 1, 8 and 15 days after tumor cell inoculation. The median survival time of animals bearing carcinoma EO 771 was significantly prolonged but multiple treatment was not more effective than a single administration of the polymer. In comparison, treatment with pyran copolymer (average mol. wt 30 000) in a similar regimen showed a very similar result. The increase of the dose to 100 mg kg^{-1} and the same treatment regimen did not prolong the median survival of the animals (Fig. 6.10.).

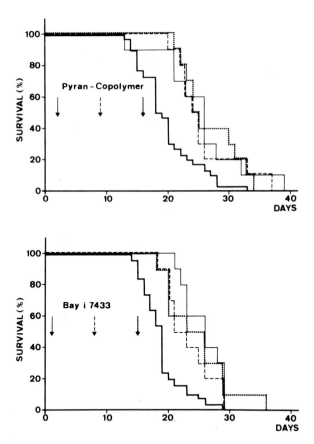

Fig. 6.9. Survival of carcinoma EO 771-bearing animals after one (——— 2 days after tumor transplantation (TT), two (– – – – 2 and 8 days after TT), and three (. . . . 2, 8 and 15 days after TT) intramuscular injections of 25 mg kg^{-1} Pyran copolymer (upper panel) or Bay i 7433 (lower panel). ——— non treated controls.

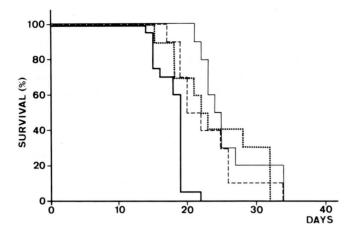

Fig. 6.10. Survival of carcinoma EO 771-bearing animals. Same treatment regimen as in Fig. 9 with 100 mg kg^{-1} Bay i 7433.

Combination of tumor excision and treatment with the polymer resulted in a retardation or inhibition of tumor recurrence. This occurred when Bay i 7433 was given either prior to, simultaneously with or after tumor surgery. Tumor excision and a single administration of different doses (5, 25 and 100 mg kg^{-1}) of the compound 6 days prior to excision of carcinoma EO 771 resulted in an increase of the survival time (Fig. 6.11.); 30–40% of the animals survived a period of 6 months. Dose dependence of the percentage of surviving animals or prolongation of survival cannot be recognized. Combination of tumor surgery and multiple treatment with the polymer are in progress.

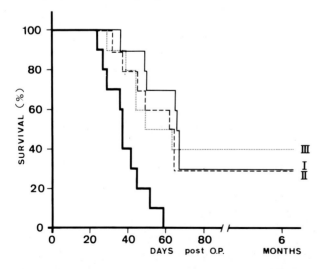

Fig. 6.11. Increase of survival time after excision of the primary carcinoma EO 771 tumors and a single intramuscular administration of different doses of Bay i 7433 6 days prior to tumor surgery.

6.3. INVESTIGATIONS INTO THE MODE OF ACTION OF BAY i 7433

Bay i 7433 does not exhibit cytostatic or cytotoxic effects in vitro on different tumor cell lines, normal mouse peritoneal cells, mouse fibroblasts or mouse spleen cells in concentrations up to 1 mg ml^{-1}. Concentrations higher than 1 mg ml^{-1} in the cell culture medium resulted in a dose-dependent decrease of [^{3}H]thymidine incorporation into the cells of fibrosarcoma FIO 26 and carcinoma EO 771 reaching background levels at a concentration of 10 mg ml^{-1}.

The polymer was not immunogenic when administered to rabbits together with complete Freund's adjuvant in several immunization cycles. Similarly, Bay i 7433 did not induce anaphylaxis in guinea pigs after subcutaneous application of 1 – 100 mg kg^{-1} 1 – 10 times on consecutive days with and without complete Freund's adjuvant.

There is no evidence that the polymer activates classical immune mechanisms. The compound did not exhibit mitogenic activity in normal mouse spleen cells, and also did not modify the response of lymphocytes to mitogens such as LPS and Con A. The humoral immune response to sheep red blood cells was neither influenced in vivo as assessed by the Jerne plaque assay nor in vitro in the Mishell–Dutton system. Accordingly, an adjuvantive effect in mice pre-treated with killed Herpes virus and Bay i 7433 was not observed after challenge with live Herpes virus. The compound also did not enhance cellular cytotoxicity of spleen cells from C57 Bl/6 mice after immunization with allogeneic YAC cells or with syngeneic Lewis lung tumor cells (P. Koldowski, personal communication). This is consistent with our observations that Bay i 7433 also exhibits anti-tumor activity in athymic Balb/c (nu/nu) mice.

The phagocytic activity of the RES was measured after ip and iv administration of 0.5 – 100 mg kg^{-1} Bay i 7433 in normal mice. The polymer neither enhanced nor inhibited carbon clearance. The compound did not enhance or inhibit phagocytosis of latex particles into peritoneal macrophages. It was also not active as a primer of the tumor necrosis factor instead of BCG.

Bay i 7433 did not induce any changes of hematocrit, bone marrow cellularity, spleen weight, or growth of erythropoietic (CFU-E) or granulopoietic (CFU-C) colonies on days 3, 5, 8, 11 and 14 after administration of 0.5 – 100 mg kg^{-1} into normal Balb/c mice.

Im administration of 5 and 50 mg kg^{-1} Bay i 7433 into CF$_1$ mice prior to challenge with EMC virus did not result in the elicitation of type 1 (day 1) or type 2 (days 4, 7, 10) interferon. The median survival times and the mortality rates were the same in the treated and the non-treated control groups.

There is no evidence that the polymer has any influence on the blood clotting systems of rats.

6.4. STUDIES ON THE EXCRETION OF THE COMPOUND

Bay i 7433 can be quantitated in body fluids after a chromatographic separation step by complexing it with iodine. Iodine reacts thereby in aqueous solution through addition to the double bonds of a few remaining vinyl bridges. This leads to a brown-reddish precipitate which is soluble in methanol/hydrochloric acid and can be quantitated photometrically at 430 nm. At least 90% of the compound is recovered by this method.

Excretion of Bay i 7433 after intravenous administration of 8 mg kg^{-1} has been investigated in Wistar rats. About 70% of the compound could be recovered from the urine in the first 4 h after injection. About 25% of the polymer were excreted between 4 and 8 h, and about 5% were found between 8 and 24 h after administration. From 24 to 48 h and from 48 h to 72 h only about 1% each of the applied dose was determined. Thus at least 95% of the polymer is excreted in the urine of rats within 24 h following application. However, these results do not exclude that minor amounts of the polymer remain in the body over longer periods of time. The excretion pattern was similar when the compound was administered intramuscularly.

Preliminary investigations with thin layer chromatography (aluminum oxide as the solid phase) provide evidence that Bay i 7433 is excreted unchanged in its chemical structure.

The kinetics of the polymer in the blood and its excretion in other animal species are presently under investigation.

6.5. STUDIES OF ACUTE AND SUBCHRONIC TOXICITY

Acute toxicity of Bay i 7433 was studied in mice, rats, rabbits, dogs and rhesus monkeys. Mice and rats tolerated 10 mg kg^{-1} after oral administration and 5 g kg^{-1} after intraperitoneal application. Intramuscularly, rats tolerated 2 g kg^{-1} Bay i 7433 without signs of adverse reactions. The LD$_{50}$ after intravenous application of the polymer into rats was determined to be 4.3 and 5.2 g kg^{-1} in female and male rats, respectively. Mice tolerated 5 g kg^{-1} of the compound given by the intravenous route. The intravenously applied polymer caused in all animals reduced motility, tonic spasms, respiratory distress, cyanosis and morphine tail. Surviving animals were symptom free within 24 h. Intravenous application of 5 g kg^{-1} Bay i 7433 to rabbits resulted in opisthotonus, tonic cramps, respiratory distress and exophthalmus. These symptoms disappeared within 1 h after injection. All animals survived the treatment.

These symptoms which only occurred after intravenous administration are probably due to the physico-chemical properties of the relatively viscous polymer solution rather than to inherent toxic properties of the compound.

Dogs, which received 2 g kg^{-1} Bay i 7433 exhibited symptoms typical for the release of endogenous histamine. The animals were again symptom free 30 min after intravenous injection of the polymer, and all animals survived the treatment. Since there is no evidence for immunogenicity of Bay i 7433 and since these anaphylactoid reactions occurred already after the first injection of the polymer, it is highly suggestive that the histamine release is non-specific i.e. that it is not mediated by specific immune mechanisms as in type I allergic reactions. The animals tolerated 5 g kg^{-1} by the oral route without any signs of adverse reactions.

Dissection of the animals after a preceding observation period of 14 days did not reveal any pathological changes.

Intraperitoneal application of Bay i 7433 daily for 3 months to rats results in dose-dependent degenerations of the proximal tubulus epithelium of the kidney. Crystal-like inclusions were observed in tubulus cells of rats which had received 300 and 1000 mg kg^{-1}. Observation of these animals, and haematological and clinical-chemical parameters did not reveal any changes which could be correlated with the application of the polymer.

Daily intravenous administration of Bay i 7433 in doses of 50, 200 and 800 mg kg^{-1} for three months into dogs did not result in any changes of haematological and clinical-chemical parameters, except in one animal each of the dose groups of 200 and 800 mg kg^{-1} a distinct increase of GPT was observed. All animals showed signs and symptoms of histamine release after the first injection. In two animals of the 800 mg kg^{-1} dose group, histopathological investigations revealed swollen liver cells with prominent fat-free vacuoles which were randomly distributed, and isolated liver cell necrosis. There was an indication of similar but less prominent changes in isolated hepatocytes in two animals of the group which received 200 mg kg^{-1} of the polymer.

Subchronic intravenous administration of Bay i 7433 to rhesus monkeys in doses of 50, 200 and 800 mg kg^{-1} also did not result in any changes of clinical, haematological and clinical-chemical parameters during the observation period. Histopathological investigations of the animals revealed inflammatory cellular infiltrations in the parenchymatous and connective tissues of the liver. Granuloma-like changes in the parenchymatous tissue of the liver, and a distinct proliferation of Kupffer cells were observed in 6 out of 8 animals of the 800 mg kg^{-1} dose group. Similar, but less marked changes were observed in all animals of the group which received 200 mg kg^{-1} of the polymer. Animals that received 50 mg kg^{-1} daily for 3 months did not exhibit granuloma-like changes in the liver tissues but, unlike the control group, inflammatory, mononuclear cell infiltrations were present. The extent of these infiltrations were, however, distinctly less marked compared to the groups which had received higher doses.

In summary, Bay i 7433 is well tolerated after a single administration of high dose. Intravenous application of the polymer to dogs led to anaphylactoid reactions due to a non-specific release of endogenous histamine. Subchronic administration of the compound to rats, dogs and monkeys was clinically well tolerated and no loss of animals occurred. In contrast to this, histopathological changes were observed but these do not show organotropy and have no functional correlation in the haematological and clinical-chemical parameters investigated.

6.6. SUMMARY AND CONCLUSIONS

Bay i 7433 is a very well tolerated compound which exhibits significant anti-tumor activity after a single injection either prior to, or after inoculation of cells from different tumor. This anti-tumor activity could be shown to be dose-dependent and to occur in a broad dose range. About 95% of the compound is excreted in the urine of Wistar rats within 24 h of iv and im administration.

Multiple administration of the polymer was not superior to a single administration when evaluated by tumor weight 21–25 days after tumor transplantation. A significant prolongation of the median survival time of tumor-bearing animals is achieved by a single administration of Bay i 7433 prior to or after tumor transplantation. However, multiple treatment in various regimens proved not to enhance survival time. Combination of tumor excision and treatment with the polymer resulted in a retardation or inhibition of tumor recurrences, in an increase of the median survival time, and an increase of 30–40% in survival over a period of more than 6 months.

The facts that Bay i 7433 is not cytotoxic or cytostatic, and that it displays significant anti-tumor activity when administered prior to tumor cell inoculation, strongly suggest that it exerts its activity via host-mediated control mechanisms. From the uncommonly good tolerability of the polymer, it may be assumed that the mode of action and/or the point of attack of the compound is highly selective.

The mode of action of this polymer is obscure. At present, there is certainly more information available as to what the polymer does not do than positive clues about its mode of action. We have at present no evidence that classic immune mechanisms are involved in the anti-tumor activity, and other mechanisms of tumor growth control must be assumed. Further investigations to elucidate the mode of action of Bay i 7433 are in progress.

ACKNOWLEDGEMENTS

The following colleagues have contributed to this paper: chemistry, Dres. Bömer, Wolf; biology, Dres. Bierling, Hewlett, Löbbecke, Opitz, Streissle; toxicology, Dres. Bomhard, Frank, Hoffmann, Kaliner, Mürmann, Schlüter, Vogel; pharmacokinetics, Dr. Wingender.

CHAPTER 7

Immunological properties of NPT 15392: a review

Joseph Wybran

Department of Immunology, Erasmus Hospital, Free University of Brussels, (Belgium)

7.1. INTRODUCTION

This chapter summarizes some of the properties of NPT 15392, a new synthetic drug developed in the field of immunopharmacology.

Its formula has been recently disclosed [1]. It is erythro-9-(2-hydroxy,3-nonyl)hypoxanthine. It is thus a drug derived from a purine base and as such it belongs to the family of isoprinosine (inosiplex) which possesses interesting immunomodulatory properties [2]. NPT 15392 is currently being investigated for its properties and possible influence on immunological functions.

Toxicity data have also been obtained. In animals, acute and subchronic experiments have been performed. At 500 mg kg^{-1} in acute studies, a single death was recorded in a group of 10 animals. The therapeutic index appears to be very high (probably around 1×10^6). In the subchronic assays (90 days), the only noticeable effect was a statistically significant increase in the blood glucose of female rats receiving 2.5 mg kg^{-1} compared to control values. In pure bred Beagle dogs, the only abnormal parameter was an increased bilirubin and total globulin after 90 days of treatment. These findings may perhaps be incidental.

In humans, tolerance studies have been carried out in volunteers receiving single oral doses from 0.4 mg to 35 mg of NPT 15392. The subjects were followed for a period of one month. There were no biological or physiological modifications in these subjects. The only toxic effect at the high doses was in a few patients a small and reversible hair loss (hairs in the comb) without real alopecia [1].

7.2. IN VITRO ANIMAL PROPERTIES

This section summarizes the data available on the properties of NPT 15392. At the First International Conference on Immunopharmacology (Brighton, July 1980) most of the investigators using NPT 15392 described their research [3]. The animal work and some human work has mainly been done by Hadden and his collaborators.

7.2.1. Lymphocyte stimulation [4]

Both mouse spleen and human lymphocytes increase their response to phyto-hemagglutinin and concanavalin A at doses between 0.01 and 0.1 μg ml^{-1}. Higher doses (10 μg ml^{-1}) are without effect or inhibitory. The response to antigens like *Candida* and *Staphylococcus* is also increased. The response is usually augmented only by 10 – 20% and thus this increment is less dramatic than with isoprinosine.

7.2.2. Suppressor function

Suppressor cells which inhibit the autologous Con A response of a mixed lymphocyte culture can also be induced by incubating the lymphocytes with 0.1 to 10 μg ml^{-1} of NPT 15392. This effect appears to be more important than with isoprinosine, where suppressor cells appear to be mainly blast cells.

7.2.3. Cytotoxicity [5]

NPT 15392 does not affect the ADCC or the NK function per se. However, it was reported by Goutner that NPT 15392 potentiates the action of suboptimal doses of interferon on NK function.

7.2.4. Macrophages [4]

NPT 15392 increases the macrophage proliferation induced by lymphokines in the guinea pig.

7.2.5. Induction of T cell markers [6]

Pahwa and his colleagues of the Sloan Kettering Institute have shown that NPT 15392 induces the appearance of Thy 1 positive cells in a Komuro-Boyse assay at concentrations as low as 0.01 to 1 μg ml^{-1}. This effect is similar to thymic factors and is remarkable in view of the very low concentrations used.

7.2.6. Nuclear refringence [7]

Pompidou et al. have shown that 0.1 μg of the drug affects lymphocyte nuclear refringence. This is suggestive to these researchers of lymphocyte activation.

7.3. IN VIVO ANIMAL EFFECTS

7.3.1. Antibody formation [8]

It appears that NPT 15392 (0.3 mg to 1 mg kg^{-1} given prior to or at the same time as the antigen increases the antibody formation, provided that the antigen is T cell dependent (e.g. sheep red blood cells). In contrast, using a T cell independent antigen (TNP-LPS), there was no increase in antibody formation. Of interest is that strains of mice which are unresponsive to levamisole (C57 BL/6 mouse) do not respond to NPT 15392.

7.3.2. Cytotoxicity

Both Faanes et al. [8] and Florentin (personal communication) have shown that NPT 15392 increases the NK activity using the spleen cells. Interestingly, the NK activity can decrease after 7 days and rebound a few days later.

7.3.3. Restoration of immunosuppression

Hadden's group [4] has reported significant augmentation of Con A response of mouse spleens in both normal mice or mice immunosuppressed with Friend leukemia virus. Sato and Tsurufuji [9] have also very interestingly reported that NPT 15392 can restore the suppressed immune function in a variety of tumor-bearing mice using intraperitoneal doses of 0.01 to 10 mg kg^{-1}. This restoration was noticed in sarcoma 80, L-1210, Ehrlich's carcinoma and Ehrlich's lung metastases. The effect was usually observed using a plaque-forming test or a delayed type of hypersensitivity. In contrast, no effect was detected in NF sarcoma implanted mice.

7.4. IN VITRO HUMAN STUDIES

7.4.1. Lymphocyte stimulation

As mentioned above, Hadden and co-workers have shown that NPT 15392 increases the response to phytohemagglutinin and concanavalin A. Wybran [10] has also found that the drug can enhance mixed lymphocyte response. In contrast to isoprinosine, where Wybran has shown the induction of a mitogenic helper factor, NPT 15392 does not induce the formation of such factor. It is possible that this non-induction provides an explanation for the observation that enhancement of stimulation is usually not very important (around 20%) in contrast to isoprinosine.

7.4.2. Active rosette formation [10,11]

NPT 15392 will increase the active T rosette formation using doses between 0.01 and 10 μg ml^{-1}. This effect is observed after 1 hour of incubation with the drug using washed lymphocytes. In some respects this phenomenon appears to be similar to the induction of the mouse Thy-1 marker. Preliminary data indicate that the active rosette formation phenomenon is due to the early appearance of a rosetting factor induced by NPT 15392. Indeed, supernatants of drug-treated lymphocytes possess the property of increasing the percentage of active T rosettes using 'virgin' lymphocytes (not incubated with the drug). Using other rosette systems (total T, autologous T and EAC), NPT 15392 did not modify their percentages using normal human lymphocytes.

7.4.3. Cytotoxicity

Preliminary data of Wybran and Schmerber [11] indicate that NPT 15392 increases specific T cell cytotoxicity (dose range 0.01 to 1 μg ml^{-1}) using the cytotoxic cells produced in a mixed lymphocyte culture system.

7.4.4. Polymorph neutrophils [10, 11]

Two types of experiments are highly suggestive of a stimulating activity upon neutrophils. Maxwell has found that zymosan-induced chemoluminescence is increased by the drug at doses varying between 0.001 and 10 μg ml^{-1}. Similarly we have observed that similar concentrations increase the phagocytic activity of isolated polymorph neutrophils upon yeast particles.

In a similar system, NPT 15392 only slightly enhances monocyte phagocytosis.

7.4.5. Leucocyte adherence inhibition test.

With Appelboom, we have shown that NPT 15392 increases the number of cells nonadherent to glass tubes. This test also indicates a direct action on T cells, since the loss of adherence, in this system, is due to a factor released by T cells which acts upon human neutrophils to decrease their adherence to glass.

7.5. IN VIVO HUMAN EFFECTS [10, 11]

Only preliminary data are available with the drug. In normal subjects, Riethmuller has shown that the oral ingestion of one dose varying between 0.7 mg and 35 mg increases in 80% of the cases the percentage of blood active T rosettes. Enhancement of PHA response was also observed.

In patients with various malignant solid tumors, Wybran and his co-workers have also observed changes in blood T cells. There appears to be a relation to the dose. With a unique oral dose of 0.4 mg, the percentage of blood active T rosettes will decrease in the first 24 to 48 h and then increase at 72 h.

A unique dose of 0.7 mg increases the percentage of active T rosettes at 24 and 48 h; they return to pretreatment values at 72 h. Using doses of 0.4 – 0.7 mg repeated every 2 or 3 days for 2 weeks, it was usually observed that, after 2 weeks, the percentages of both active and total T rosettes had increased. The response to PHA is not as clear cut, usually with an increment in about half the patients.

The Tumor Immunology Project Group (TIPG) is currently investigating various immunological parameters in cancer patients taking repeated doses of 0.4 mg or 0.7 mg of the drug.

7.5. DISCUSSION

All the studies concerning the new compound NPT 15392 should be considered with a very cautious interest at this time since most of the data are derived from abstracts, personal communications or personal work. Nevertheless, since most of the reports are usually confirmatory, one can start drawing the profile of the drug.

NPT 15392 appears to be a nontoxic drug with a very high therapeutic index. The active concentrations both in vitro and in vivo are very low and are probably the lowest ever described with a synthetic immunological compound.

It acts on T cells at various levels : induction of markers and differentiation (Thy 1 marker, active T rosettes), enhancement of T helper cell (T dependent antibody response) and T suppressor cell (in vitro), enhancement of T cell response to mitogens and antigens, enhancement of T cell cytotoxicity. All these actions on T cells have usually been described both in vitro and in vivo in animals and in man. Obviously, it is important to better define the optimal dose necessary to obtain these responses by carefully performing phase I and II clinical trials. The TIPG is currently attempting to define these doses.

Limited data also indicate that NPT 15392 can stimulate some macrophage function.

Interestingly and especially in the field of tumor, NPT 15392 enhances various cytotoxic functions like T cell and NK cytotoxicity.

Finally in view of its stimulatory effect upon human neutrophil functions, NPT 15392 should also be tried in various situations where such activation may appear helpful in eradicating a disease process or a functional defect.

7.7. CONCLUSIONS

NPT 15392 is an interesting immuno-modulating drug active at very low concentrations. It has shown activity in multiple systems involving pre T and T cells, macrophages and neutrophils, both in animals and in man. Current studies will better define the mode of action upon the various subsets of immune cells, especially that high doses appear to be suppressive in vitro. It has an interesting action in NK and T cell cytotoxicity. All the results indicate that it acts both in normal subjects and in immuno-suppressed subjects.

Therefore, NPT 15392 will probably very soon be investigated in such clinical conditions as cancer, where restoration or stimulation of the immune system, with careful immunological monitoring, is thought to be promising.

REFERENCES

1 Simon, L.N. Settineri, R., Pfadenhauer, E.P., Jones, C., Maxwell, K. and Glasky, A.J. NPT 15392 : A pharmacologic and toxicologic profile. Internat. J. Immunopharmacol. 2, 200, 1980.
2 Wybran, J., Appelboom, T. and Govaerts, A. Inosiplex, A stimulating agent for normal human T cells and human leucocytes. J. Immunol. 121, 1184-1187, 1978.
3 Hadden, J.W. and Wybran, J. Isoprinosine, NPT 15392 and Azimexone : modulators of lymphocyte and macrophage development and function. in Advances in Immunopharmacology (J. Hadden, P. Mullen, L. Chedid and F. Spreafico Eds, Pergamon Press; Oxford (in press).
4 Hadden, J.W., Hadden, E.M., Spira, T., and Giner-Sorolla, A., NPT 15392 : A modulator of in vitro lymphocyte and macrophage functions. Internat. J. Immunopharmacol. 2, 198, 1980.
5 Goutner, A. In vitro modulation of natural killer cell activity by isoprinosine, NPT 15392 and interferon. Internat. J. Immunopharmacol. 2, 197, 1980.
6 Pahwa, R., Ikehara, S., Hadden, J., and Good, R.A. In vitro effect of isoprinosine and an analogue (15392) on murine T cell differentiation and function. Internat. J. Immunopharmacol. 2, 199, 1980.
7 Pompidou, A., Mace, B., Esnous, D. and Mayrand, C. Early activation of human lymphocytes nuclei by isoprinosine. Internat. J. Immunopharmacol. 2, 196, 1980.
8 Faanes, R.B., Merluzzi, V.J., Walker, M., Williams, N., Ralph, P, and Hadden, J.W. Immunoenhancing activity of NPT 15392 : a potential immune response modifier. Internat. J. Immunopharmacol. 2, 197, 1980.
9 Sato, S., and Tsurufuji, M. NPT 15392 : immunorestorative effects in tumor-suppressed mice. Internat. J. Immunopharmacol, 2, 200, 1980.
10 Wybran, J. NPT 15392, a new synthetic immunomodulatory agent : human, in vitro and in vivo (cancer patients) effects. Internat. J. Immunopharmacol. 2, 201, 1980.
11 Wybran, J. and Schmerber, J. Submitted for publication.

CHAPTER 8

Immunological properties of azimexon in normal mice, aged mice and cancer patients

A. Goutner, I. Florentin, M. Bruley-Rosset and F. Nasrat

ICIG, INSERM U. 50, Hôpital Paul-Brousse, Villejuif (France)

8.1. INTRODUCTION

Inhibition of tumor growth in experimental animals by immune adjuvants has been known for many years [10].

In man, positive clinical trials have been reported but conflicting results have also been produced [15]. Part of the controversy might reside in the use of living bacteria such as *Bacillus Calmette Guérin* (BCG) or killed bacteria such as *Corynebacterium parvum* (CP). These two species of bacteria probably exhibit strain variations and their indefinite composition, the difficulty of quantifying their preparations and controlling their administration could partly be responsible for nonreproducible results. In addition, these adjuvants could induce specific and nonspecific suppressor cells leading to unfavourable clinical effects.

Thus, we are in great need of immune adjuvants with defined chemical characteristics, of reproducible administration, allowing measurement of their pharmacokinetics and possibly having restricted cellular targets. Synthetic immunomodulating substances fulfil these requirements and might represent a new development in the immunotherapy of cancer. Adverse effects such as induction of suppressor cells could be avoided because of the intrinsic properties of the immunomodulating molecule or by proper dose scheduling.

A new class of synthetic immunomodulators, the 2-cyanaziridines were introduced by Bicker et al. [2]. The first compound of this series, Imexon (or BM 06002) provoked nausea and vomiting in about 20% of the patients to whom it was administered [11]. Thus azimexon (or BM 12531) was developed in order to try to reduce these side effects. Azimexon has been reported to be able to prevent tumor growth in experimental animals [1].

We initially studied in normal immunocompetent mice the effect of a single dose of azimexon on various immunological parameters as a function of the time of administration. The influence of azimexon administration on T cells, B cells, macrophages, K cells and NK cells has been examined. This model was aimed at revealing the immunostimulatory properties of azimexon.

To follow closely the human situation, long term administration of azimexon has been studied in aging mice to reveal its immunorestorative properties and to analyze its influence on the development of spontaneous tumors, and on immune parameters.

Finally, a phase I study has been performed in immunodepressed cancer patients to reveal its potential in the restoration or the stimulation of the immune system, as studied by delayed type hypersensitivity reactions, mitogen responsiveness and spontaneous cell mediated cytotoxicity.

8.2. MATERIAL AND METHODS

Azimexon (BM 12531) was obtained from Boehringer Mannheim.

8.2.1. Mouse studies

All mice were purchased from Bomholtgard Ltd (Denmark). 2 month old female (C57 B1/6 × DBA 2) F_1 mice received a single iv injection of 500 µg of azimexon 1, 3, 7 or 10 days before immunologic testing.

C57 B1/6 female retired breeders were purchased at the age of 6 months. They received weekly ip injections of 500 µg of azimexon from 12 to 18 months of age. Control mice received weekly ip injection of saline.

All animals were inspected at least once a week and more often when they were thought to be ill. Immune testing was performed between the age of 18 and 19 months.

During the period of treatment, most dead mice or mice killed in poor conditions were necropsied and all surviving mice were killed after the age of 19 months and submitted to a pathological examination.

8.2.2. Immunological tests

All the tests have been described in detail previously [5,6].

8.2.2.1. Delayed-type hypersensitivity (DTH) reaction
Mice were sensitized by applying oxazolone to the abdomen skin. The DTH reaction was elicited 7 days later by a second application of the sensitizing agent on both ears. Ear thickness was measured just before and 24 h after the challenge.

8.2.2.2. Cytolytic T cell activity
5×10^7 spleen cells were incubated at 37°C in Falcon flasks in the presence or in the

absence of mitomycin-treated P815 tumor cells for 4 days. The RPMI 1640 culture medium contained antibiotics, glutamine and 5×10^{-5} Ml mercaptoethanol (ME) was added or not. After 4 days of culture, the suspensions were centrifuged and the number of viable cells enumerated. Various numbers of spleen cells were incubated in U-shaped microplates for 4 h at 37°C in the presence of 1×10^4 ^{51}Cr-labelled P815 tumor cells, the effector to target cell ratio varying from 30:1 to 3:1. The amount of chromium released in the supernatants was measured in a gamma counter. Cultures were done in triplicate and the percentage of specific lysis was calculated as for NK activity but spontaneous release was obtained by the mean of lysis of cultures containing 1×10^4 ^{51}Cr-labelled P815 as target and varying numbers of spleen cells cultivated in the absence of P815 tumor cells.

8.2.2.3. Spleen cell response to mitogens: suppressor cell detection

Spleen cells from agent-treated or from control mice were cultivated in microplates (5×10^5 cells/0.2 ml) for 52 h in the presence of an optimal dose of phytohemagglutinin (PHA; Wellcome Laboratories) or lipopolysaccharide (LPS ; Difco). The cultures were pulsed with 1 μCi tritiated thymidine ([^{3}H]TdR; specific activity 25 Ci mmol^{-1}; CEA; France) for the last 4 h of incubation, at the end of which the cells were collected and processed for radioactivity counting. For detection of suppressor cells, 5×10^5 spleen cells from normal mice were stimulated by the mitogens in the presence of 2.5×10^5 spleen cells from agent-treated mice. The proliferative response of the mixed cultures was compared with that of parallel cultures of 7.5×10^5 normal spleen cells.

8.2.2.4. Antibody-forming cell response

Mice were immunized intraperitoneally with either 300 μg trinitrophenylated hemocyanin (TNP-KLH) or 0.3 μg trinitrophenylated lipopolysaccharide (TNP-LPS). The number of IgM plaque-forming cells (PFC) in the spleen was determined by the method described by Cunningham and Szenberg, by using TNP-coated sheep erythrocytes as indicator cells.

8.2.2.5. Assay for macrophage-mediated cytostasis

The in vitro cytostatic activity of peritoneal macrophages was determined by using the tritiated thymidine ([^{3}H]TdR) incorporation test [4]. In order to avoid competition with unlabelled thymidine released by activated macrophages, tumor cells, after 18 h of incubation in the presence of macrophages, were harvested, washed, diluted in fresh medium (RPMI 1640) and redistributed in a new microplate II. 1 μCi per well of [^{3}H]TdR was then added for the last 4 h of culture and thymidine incorporated into tumor cells was measured in a B counter. Results are expressed as mean cpm of [^{3}H]TdR incorporation $\pm$ standard error of six cultures and as percentage inhibition of tumor cell proliferation.

8.2.2.6. Antibody-dependent cellular cytotoxicity (ADCC)

Various numbers of spleen cells from agent-treated or from control mice were incubated in microplates for 17 h with 10^4 ^{51}Cr-labelled chick red blood cells

(CRBC) and in the presence of a 1:20 000 final dilution of rabbit anti-CRBC serum. The effector/target cell ratios varied from 100:1 to 12:1. The percentage of specific lysis was calculated by using the equation:

$$\% \text{ lysis} = \frac{\text{experimental release} - \text{spontaneous release}}{\text{maximal release} - \text{spontaneous release}} \times 100$$

Results were also expressed in terms of lytic units (LU_{50}) with one LU_{50} defined as the number of spleen cells required to give 50% specific lysis. The number of LU_{50}/spleen was calculated.

8.2.2.7. Natural killer cell activity

Various numbers of spleen cells were incubated for 4 h at 37°C with 10^4 ^{51}Cr-labelled YAC-1 lymphoma cells in U-shaped microplates. The effector to target cell ratio varied from 200:1 to 25:1. The amount of ^{51}Cr released in the supernatants was measured in a gamma counter. Cultures were done in triplicate and the percentage of specific lysis was calculated as above. Spontaneous release was obtained by the mean of lysis in six cultures containing 10^4 ^{51}Cr-labelled YAC-1 cells as targets and 10^6 thymus cells as negative effectors.

8.2.2. Human studies

Patients bearing advanced solid tumors were skin tested for seven recall antigens (tuberculin, candidin, trycophytin, tetanus toxoid, diphtheria toxoid, proteus extract, streptococci extract. Multitest system provided by Institut Mérieux). Anergic or hypoergic patients (outside the normal range determined on 830 normal subjects) [13] and without any treatment for at least one month were eligible for this study. 200 mg of azimexon were administered iv or per os three days per week for two weeks. Three days after the last administration of azimexon skin tests were performed. In addition, seven breast cancer patients without a perceptible tumor but anergic or hypoergic several months after surgery and/or radiotherapy, were submitted to the same protocol.

8.2.2.1. Mitogen stimulation

Mononuclear cells were isolated from heparinized venous blood by flotation on Ficoll metrizoate, and cultured in microplates in 0.2 ml of RPMI 1640 supplemented with 20% of AB serum, 25 mM Hepes, 10 mg % glutamine. They were stimulated for four days with PHA (Difco, 0.9 and 0.18 µg per well), and tetradecanoyl phorbol acetate-TPA (Consolidated Midland, N.Y., 200 and 20 ng per well). Cell concentration was 10^5 per well for PHA stimulation and 2×10^5 in the case of TPA. Six hours before the end of the incubation 0.4 µCi of tritiated thymidine (CEA-France) was added to each well. The culture was harvested with an automated harvester (Mash I, Microbiological Associates). The incorporated [^{3}H]thymidine was measured with a Packard Tricarb scintillation counter. Results are expressed as the mean of triplicate determinations ± standard error.

8.2.2.2. Spontaneous cell-mediated cytotoxicity

NK cell activity of mononuclear cells was measured on ^{51}Cr-labelled K562 target cells in a 3.5 h assay. The test was performed in U-shaped Linbro microplates (Flow Laboratories) with 10^4 target cells per well and varying numbers of effector cells in a total volume of 250 μl. The assay was performed in RPMI supplemented with 20% human AB serum. The supernatants were harvested with the Titertek collection system (Flow laboratories) and counted in a Packard gamma counter. Maximal lysis was determined by adding detergent to the target cells and spontaneous release by incubation in the absence of effector cells.

The percentage of specific cytotoxicity was calculated as follows:

$$\% \text{ cytoxicity} = \frac{\text{experimental} - \text{spontaneous release}}{\text{maximal} - \text{spontaneous release}} \times 100$$

All groups were done in triplicate and the results are expressed as mean ± standard deviation.

8.3. RESULTS

8.3.1. Immunological effect of a single injection of azimexon in normal immunocompetent mice.

8.3.1.1. Delayed type hypersensitivity reaction

As shown in Table 8.I, azimexon when injected 1, 3, 7 or 10 days before contact sensitization with oxazolone, is able to increase the intensity of the DTH reaction as evaluated by ear thickness measurements. No enhancing effect was observed when azimexon was administered on day 0 at the same time as oxazolone.

Table 8.I.

Effect of azimexon administration on delayed-type hypersensitivity to oxazolone

Day of azimexon injection before sensitization	Mean ear thickness increment (± S.E., in 0.01 mm units)	Relative response
0	7.50 ± 1.24	1.2
−1	11.10 ± 0.86*	1.8
−3	10.40 ± 0.91*	1.7
−7	9.70 ± 0.51*	1.5
−10	9.80 ± 0.44*	1.6
Controls	6.25 ± 0.50	

Mice were sensitized with oxazolone on day 0 and challenged on both ears 7 days later. Ear thickness was measured just before and 24 h after the challenge.

* The response of the treated mice is significantly different from the control response.

8.3.1.2. Cytotoxic T cell activity

Fig. 8.1 shows that azimexon enhanced the generation of cytotoxic T cell against P815 target cell when administered in vivo 1 or 7 days before the in vitro culture of spleen cells.

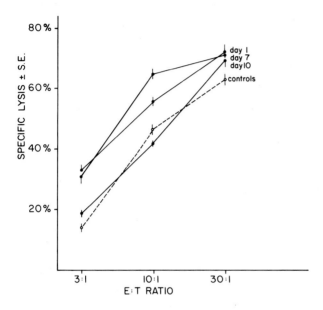

Fig. 8.1.   Influence of azimexon administered 1, 7 or 10 days before testing on the in vitro generation of cytolytic T cells in young mice.

8.3.1.3. Antibody response

Mice were immunized either with a thymus dependent (TNP-KLH) or a thymus-independent antigen (TNP-LPS). Table 8.II shows that azimexon was able to significantly potentiate the anti-TNP response when injected 1, 3, 7 or 10 days before TNP-KLH. No potentiation was observed after the simultaneous administration of azimexon and TNP-KLH.

The antibody response to the thymus-independent antigen was also significantly enhanced when azimexon was administered 1, 3, 7 or 10 days before TNP-LPS, as shown in Table 8.III. Again, simultaneous administration of azimexon and TNP-LPS did not result in any effect.

8.3.1.4. Macrophage cytostatic activity

Table 8.IV shows that azimexon is able to render peritoneal macrophages cytostatic for L-1210 leukemic cells when administered at least 7–10 days before testing.

In contrast, 3 days after Azimexon injection peritoneal macrophages did not exhibit any increase in cytostatic activity.

Table 8.II.

Effect of azimexon administration on the antibody response to a thymus-dependent antigen (TNP-KLH)

Day of azimexon injection	Mean No. anti-TNP-PFC/spleen (±S.E.)	Relative response
0	3028 ± 311	1.0
−1	4700 ± 316*	1.9
−3	3731 ± 171*	1.5
−7	4369 ± 146*	1.7
−10	5672 ± 216*	2.3
Controls (antigen alone on day 0)	2506 ± 180	

Mice were immunized with 300 μg TNP-KLH in saline and the plaque-forming cells (PFC) were counted in the spleen 5 days later.

* The response of the treated mice is significantly different from the control response.

8.3.1.5. Spleen cell response to mitogens

As illustrated in Fig.8.2. a slight but significant decrease of the proliferative response to the T cell mitogen PHA was detected from days 1 to 10 after azimexon administration. The response to the B cell mitogen was more markedly depressed but only from days 1 to 7.

Table 8.III.

Effect of azimexon administration on the antibody response to a thymus-independent antigen (TNP-LPS)

Day of azimexon injection	Mean No. of anti-TNP-PFC/spleen (± S.E.)	Relative response
0	178 880 ± 11 109	0.8
−1	461 630 ± 13 932*	2.2
−3	288 380 ± 15 996*	1.3
−7	456 500 ± 14 039*	2.1
−10	364 860 ± 11 706*	1.7
Controls (antigen alone on day 0)	213 000 ± 6 700	

Mice were immunized with 0.3 μg TNP-LPS in saline and the plaque-forming cells were counted in the spleen 3 days later.

* The response of the treated mice is significantly different from the control response.

Table 8.IV.

Effect of azimexon on macrophage cytostatic activity on L-1210 leukemic cells

Agent	Day of administration		
	3	7	10
Azimexon	0%[a]	50%	65%

[a]Cytostatic index $= 100 - \dfrac{[^3H]TdR \text{ incorporation by tumor cells exposed to agent-treated macrophages}}{[^3H]TdR \text{ incorporation by tumor cells exposed to normal macrophages}} \times 100.$

This depression of T and B cell responsiveness to mitogen stimulation could result from the induction of suppressor cells. To test this possibility spleen cells from azimexon-treated mice were cocultured with normal spleen cells in the

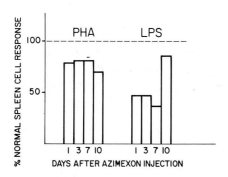

Fig. 8.2.   Mitogen responsiveness of azimexon-treated young mice, expressed as a percentage of the normal response.

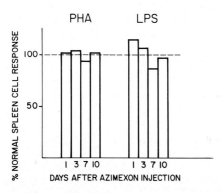

Fig. 8.3.   Effect of spleen cells from azimexon-treated young mice on the mitogen responsiveness of spleen cells from normal animals, expressed as a percentage of the control response.

presence of PHA or LPS. As shown in Fig. 8.3 no suppressive activity could be detected in the spleen of azimexon-treated mice at any time after agent administration.

8.3.1.6. Antibody dependent cell mediated cytotoxicity
As shown in Table 8.V, azimexon administered 1, 3 or 14 days before testing induced a decrease in the lytic capacity of spleen cells, using antibody-coated chicken red blood cells as targets. Lytic activity was reduced on a per cell basis as well as per spleen.

8.3.1.7. Spontaneous cell mediated cytotoxicity
Azimexon, as shown in Fig. 8.4 induced a maximal stimulation of splenic NK cell activity when administered three days before testing.

Table 8.V.

Effect of azimexon on the antibody-dependent cellular cytotoxicity against antibody-coated chick erythrocytes

Agent	Day of administration	LU_{50} value ($\times 10^4$)	No. LU/spleen
Azimexon	1	23	220
	3	30.5	240
	14	32	210
(Controls)	–	12.5	460

8.3.2. Long-term administration of azimexon in aging mice

After a 6-month treatment of weekly injections of azimexon or saline, the mice which at that time were between the age of 18 and 19 months were killed and various immunological parameters of potential anti-tumor efficacy were determined.

8.3.2.1. Macrophage-mediated cytostasis
The cytostatic activity of peritoneal macrophages for tumor cell is summarized in . Control aged mice showed a decreased activity compared to young mice. In contrast, azimexon-treated mice presented at least the same level of cytostatic activity as young mice. The interference of unlabelled thymidine released by macrophages was avoided by the transfer of the tumor target cells in fresh medium into new microplates without effector cells before adding [^{3}H]TdR.

8.3.2.2. Natural killer cell activity
Splenic NK cell activity is very strongly depressed by age, as has been described by others [7]. As shown in Fig. 8.5, 18 month old control mice had a very low level of

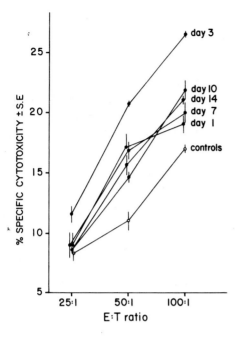

Fig. 8.4. The effect of azimexon administered 1, 3, 7, 10, 14 days before in vitro testing of NK cell activity.

Table 8.VI.

Peritoneal macrophage cytostatic activity against tumor cells of young untreated or aged treated or untreated mice

| | Age of mice: | 2 months | 18 months | 18 months |
	Mice treated with:	untreated	untreated	azimexon
[^{3}H]TdR incorporation into tumor cells (cpm ± S.E.)		8660 ± 685	28 664 ± 1061	4923 ± 236
Inhibition[a] of tumor cell proliferation (%)		70% *P*<0.01	–	83% *P*<0.01

[a] % inhibition = $\dfrac{\text{mean number of [}^3\text{H]TdR cpm incorporated into tumor cells in presence of macrophages from young untreated or aged treated mice}}{\text{mean number of [}^3\text{H]TdR cpm incorporated into tumor cells in presence of macrophages from untreated aged mice}}$

spontaneous cell-mediated cytotoxicity. In azimexon-treated mice, NK activity was even more depressed.

8.3.2.3. Antibody-dependent, cell-mediated cytotoxicity

K cell cytotoxic activity for chicken red blood cells coated with specific rabbit antibodies was elevated in aging mice. Azimexon does not modify this activity.

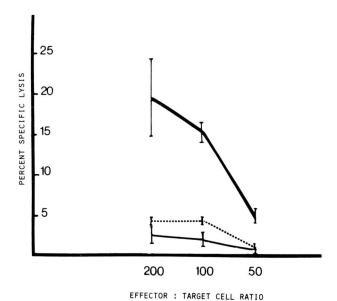

Fig. 8.5. Splenic NK cell activity of untreated old mice (– – –), azimexon-treated old mice (——) and young mice (——).

8.3.2.4. Cytolytic T cell activity

The capacity of spleen cells to generate cytotoxic T cells after in vitro allogeneic stimulation has been tested in the absence or in the presence of 2-mercaptoethanol (2-ME). Makinodan [9] has shown that 2-ME was able to enhance the in vitro primary antibody formation of old spleen cells much more than the one of young spleen cells. As shown in Fig. 8.6. 2-ME was also especially effective in maintaining the cytotoxic ability of T splenic T cells of aged mice. A slight efficacy of azimexon was only observed in the absence of 2-ME and at the effector to target cell ratio of 30/1.

8.3.2.5. Mortality of the animals during the treatment and development of spontaneous tumors

At the time of testing the survival of the mice was similar in the two groups (40% mortality).

As shown in Table 8.VII, six out of 27 (22%) untreated old mice had a malignant tumor compared to three out of 30 in the azimexon-treated group. This difference is not statistically significant. However, it should be noted that none of the mice receiving azimexon developed a lymphoma, versus four out of 27 in the control group.

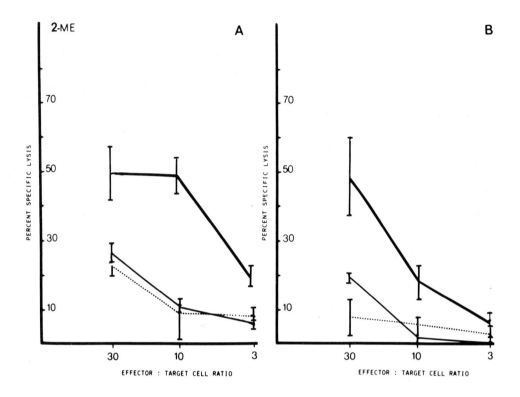

Fig. 8.6. Generation of cytotoxic T-cells from spleen cells of untreated old mice (– – –), azimexon-treated old mice (——) and young mice (——) in the presence (A) or absence of 2-mercaptoethanol (B).

8.3.3. Effect of azimexon administration in immunodepressed cancer patients

Sixteen patients bearing various solid tumors and seven breast cancer patients received azimexon, which was perfectly tolerated.

Table 8.VIII gives the histological diagnosis of the first 16 patients and shows the effect of azimexon on their DTH reactions. A restoration of DTH reactions was obtained in 11 out of 16 cases.

Six out of the seven immunodepressed breast cancer patients were also restored, as shown in Table 8.IX.

Mitogen responsiveness was studied in 12 of the patients bearing advanced solid tumors. Tables 8.X. and 8.XI. show, respectively, the results obtained in the five patients who remained anergic and in the seven patients who were restored after azimexon administration. It can be seen that, before azimexon treatment, the TPA responsiveness is depressed in eight out of 12 cases while the PHA responsiveness is abnormal in only four cases.

After azimexon administration in the five patients remaining anergic, the

Table 8.VII.

Incidence and histological types of spontaneous tumors: effect of different treatments

Group of mice	Histological form of the tumors developed in aged mice	Tumors (%)[a]	P (compared to untreated aged mice)
Untreated aged mice (27 mice)	1 adenocarcinoma (genital tract) 1 undifferentiated malignant lymphoma (spleen) 1 undifferentiated malignant lymphoma (lymph node) 1 immunoblastic lymphoma (lymph node) 1 adenocarcinoma (lung) 1 malignant lymphoma unclassified (spleen)	6/27 = 22%	
Azimexon-treated mice (30 mice)	1 squamous cell carcinoma (skin) 1 adenocarcinoma (skin appendage) 1 undifferentiated carcinoma (lung)	3/30 = 10%	0.10<P<0.20

[a]% of tumors = $\dfrac{\text{number of tumor-bearing mice}}{\text{total number of mice in the group}}$.

proliferative response to TPA was either abolished, or deeply depressed as in the patient who had a normal reactivity to TPA before azimexon administration. In contrast all the seven restored patients had normal TPA responses after azimexon administration. In four of them the level of reactivity was clearly abnormal before azimexon administration (patients Nos 7, 11, 12 and 15). In one case the PHA responsiveness was not simultaneously restored (patient 12).

Table 8.XII shows the effect of azimexon on the spontaneous cell mediated cytotoxicity of eight patients (six patients bearing solid tumors, two breast cancer patients).

In two cases the NK activity continued to decline. These two patients did not exhibit a restoration of their DTH reaction. In the six remaining cases the NK activity rose after azimexon administration. The NK activity of patients 5 and 6, which was normal at the start, reached a high level after azimexon application, comparable to the stimulation that we observed in interferon treated patients.

8.4. DISCUSSION

The effects of a single injection of 500 µg of azimexon to normal mice have clearly demonstrated its immunomodulating properties. Azimexon potentiated the antibody response to TNP-LPS, a thymus-independent antigen, implicating a direct action on B cells. Azimexon was also able to enhance T cell functions. The DTH

Table 8.VIII.

The effect of azimexon (B.M.) on the DTH reaction of anergic cancer patients

Patient's diagnosis	Before azimexon	After azimexon
1. Colon carcinoma	0	0
2. Cervix carcinoma	0	0
3. Nasopharyngeal carcinoma	0	0
4. Breast carcinoma	0	0
5. Breast carcinoma	0	0
6. Breast carcinoma	0	T = 2 mm S = 3 mm C = 3 mm
7. Bronchus carcinoma	T = 2 mm C = 2 mm	T = 3 mm D = 2 mm C = 3 mm TR = 2 mm TET= 2 mm
8. Bronchus carcinoma	0	C = 3 mm
9. Bronchus carcinoma	0	TR = 2 mm TET = 2 mm S = 2 mm C = 2 mm
10. Liposarcoma	0	TR = 3 mm C = 3 mm
11. Cervix carcinoma	0	S = 2 mm D = 2 mm
12. Hodgkin's disease	0	C = 2 mm TR = 3 mm
13. Squamous carcinoma	0	T = 3 mm
14. Melanoma	0	T = 6 mm
15. Renal carcinoma	0	T = 4 mm
16. Ovary carcinoma	0	T = 3mm

C = candidin; S = streptococci extract; T = tuberculin; TR = tetanus toxoid; TET = trycophytin; D = diphtheria toxoid; DTH c14 delayed type hypersensitivity.

Table 8.IX.

The effect of azimexon on the DTH reaction of immunodepressed breast cancer patients

Patient	Before azimexon	After azimexon
1	0	0
2	0	T = 2 mm TR = 2 mm
3	0	C = 2 mm TR = 5 mm
4	0	T = 2 mm
5	0	T = 2 mm C = 2 mm TR = 2 mm
6	TR = 3 mm	TR = 5 mm C = 2 mm
7	0	T = 3 mm

C = candidin; T = tuberculin; TR = trycophytin

reactions to oxazolone were increased, as well as the generation of cytotoxic T cells, the antibody response to a thymus-dependent antigen. However, these T cell effector mechanisms are dependent on monocytes or macrophages. Transfer experiments are needed to establish whether azimexon acted in these instances directly on T cell or indirectly on macrophages or both.

Indeed, it was shown that azimexon could strongly activate the cytostatic

Table 8.X.

Azimexon influence on mitogen responsiveness

Patient diagnosis	Before azimexon					After azimexon				
	PHA$_1$	PHA$_2$	TPA$_1$	TPA$_2$	DTH	PHA$_1$	PHA$_2$	TPA$_1$	TPA$_2$	DTH
1. Colon carcinoma	51 799	19 506	906	550	–	31 853	28 870	1 497	1 054	–
2. Cervix carcinoma	11 228	1 368	21 333	23 820	–	1 945	534	4 038	2 557	–
3. Nasopharyngeal carcinoma	5 198	1 406	1 262	1 585	–	1 276	195	366	304	–
4. Breast cancer	61 121	3 100	2 302	2 637	–	41 864	6 001	679	635	–
5. Breast cancer	12 517	1 985	8 898	4 410		N.D.	5 814	N.D.	935	

PHA = phytohemagglutinin; TPA = tetradecanoyl phorbol acetate; DTH = delayed type hypersensitivity; N.D. = not done

Table 8.XI.

Azimexon influence on mitogen responsiveness

Patient diagnosis	Before azimexon					After azimexon				
	PHA$_1$	PHA$_2$	TPA$_1$	TPA$_2$	DTH	PHA$_1$	PHA$_2$	TPA$_1$	TPA$_2$	DTH
7. Bronchus carcinoma	39 650	17 732	4 590	3 759	–	50 213	6 108	18 664	13 300	+
8. Bronchus carcinoma	43 079	6 039	38 891	33 289	–	20 621	23 037	17 776	37 440	+
11. Cervix carcinoma	79 373	13 716	1 665	1 232	–	75 585	33 241	55 803	57 673	+
12. Hodgkin's disease	1 273	1 416	5 632	3 060	–	2 064	4 847	4 118	17 709	+
14. Melanoma	52 692	36 012	31 141	17 977	–	46 114	25 323	32 201	37 057	+
15. Renal carcinoma	86 069	13 579	6 533	609	–	49 302	6 513	24 549	23 350	+
16. Ovarian carcinoma	93 352	27 169	31 659	32 727	–	46 349	2 831	43 620	31 581	+

PHA = phytohemagglutinin; TPA = tetradecanoyl phorbol acetate; DTH = delayed type hypersensitivity.

Table 8.XII.

Influence of azimexon on spontaneous cell-mediated cytotoxicity (K 562 target cells)

Patient		Effector/target cell ratio					
		100/1	75/1	50/1	25/1	12.5/1	5/1
1.	Before	47.5±1.2%	46.9±5.2%	41.8±1.7%	42.9±2.2%	29.8±1.7%	13.8±0.9%
	After	52.9±1.8%	52.2±4.4%	49.6±1.5%	43.4±0.2%	33.1±3%	26.1±2.4%
2.	Before	30.8±2.8%	21.4±7%	20.8±3.6%	21.1±0.8%	13.8±7%	6.9±2.3%
	After	51 ±6.5%	49.6±3.8%	41 ±3.5%	28.5±1.6%	18.5±2%	11.8±1.1%
3.	Before	29 ±1.5%	ND	37 ±2.1%	31 ±1%	ND	ND
	After	34 ±3.4%	ND	46 ±1%	42 ±3%	ND	ND
4.	Before	43.2±5.8%	ND	45.5±3.3%	41 ±0.1%	25.2±1.7%	ND
	After	44 ±2.7%	ND	46.3±1.1%	42.4±1%	41.2±1.4%	22.3±1%
5.	Before	44 ±5.8%	40.5±1.8%	35.7±1%	28 ±1.1%	ND	ND
	After	79.8±2.4%	74.4±3.9%	71.1±4.3%	60 ±9%	53 ±1.1%	30.7±3.5%
6.	Before	48.3±0.7%	50.7±2%	48.3±4.1%	36.5±1.9%	21.2±1.1%	7.4±1.3%
	After	69.5±5.3%	56.5±3.8%	ND	41.4±9.5%	28 ±2.4%	24 ±2.3%
7.	Before	36 ±1%	ND	24.3±2.7%	13.7±4.6%	9.7±1.2%	4.8±0.7%
	After	24.7±2.1%	ND	11.2±1.9%	10.3±1.6%	6.8±0.6%	3.9±0.3%
8.	Before	45.4±0.3%	40.9±0.7%	33.9±5%	22.7±1%	ND	8.9±3.1%
	After	33.9±2.5%	28.8±1%	21 ±0.3%	14.8±2.3%	7.8±1.1%	3.7±0.9%

N.D. = not done

capacity of macrophages for tumor cells. Azimexon was also able to activate another type of cell endowed with antitumor potential: the NK cell. In contrast, ADCC activity was depressed after azimexon administration.

The results obtained in aged mice cannot be directly compared to those of young mice since the modality of administration of azimexon and the immune status of the animals are different. However, some common traits have been recorded.

Aged control mice exhibited, compared to young mice, a severe impairment of the generation of cytotoxic T cells, of macrophage activation as measured by the inhibition of tumor cell proliferation, and of NK cell activity. On the other hand, antibody-dependent, cell-mediated cytotoxicity was elevated in aged mice.

Azimexon was able to stimulate slightly the generation of CTL and to increase further on the elevation of ADCC activity. The depression of NK cell activity was slightly accentuated, but only the splenic compartment has been studied. The most noticeable impact of azimexon on the immune system of aged mice was on the macrophage. Macrophage inhibition of tumor cell proliferation was completely abolished in untreated aged mice. Aged mice receiving azimexon exhibited a level of cytostatic macrophage activity superior to that of fully immunocompetent young mice. The decrease of the incidence of spontaneous tumor in the azimexon-treated animals, although not statistically significant, could be explained by this restoration of the macrophage cytostatic activity.

Human studies have revealed the powerful effect of azimexon on the DTH reactions, which consisted of the restoration of a normal reactivity in anergic or hypoergic patients and not of the stimulation of a competent immune system as in the mouse. This action on the DTH reactions is probably of therapeutic importance since anergic patients have a worse prognosis than reactive ones [12].

This potent influence of azimexon is further strengthened by the in vitro proliferative response of T lymphocytes to TPA, which is the selective mitogen of the T cells forming active rosettes [16].

In this study, patients exhibiting positive DTH reactions after azimexon administration all had a normal in vitro response to TPA. Thus the T cells responding to TPA in vitro might represent one of the subpopulations of cells necessary to express in vivo delayed-type hypersensitivity reactions and could be the cellular targets of azimexon. In fact, Boerner et al. [3] have shown that azimexon given to cancer patients can augment the percentage of active E rosettes. However, as in the mouse, these T cell functions are dependent on monocytes and azimexon could also stimulate T cells via macrophages.

In humans, azimexon is also able to restore or to enhance NK cell activity. Although our patients were relatively old their NK cell activity was not abolished, as it had been in aged mice. This is an important species difference already noted by several authors [7]. This effect of azimexon on human NK cells might be important since they seem to be mostly active against the development of metastasis [14], which is the main cause of death in cancer patients.

Thus, azimexon could be used not only as an immunorestorative substance but also as a compound exhibiting an immunotherapeutic potential. In fact, azimexon has already induced tumor regression in a few patients [8].

ACKNOWLEDGEMENTS

The work of the authors described here was supported partially by contracts DGRST No. 78 7 2651 and INSERM C.L. No. 78 5 16 82

REFERENCES

1   Bicker, U. Immunomodulating effects of BM 12531 in animals and tolerance in man. Cancer Treat. Rep. 62, 1987-1996, 1978.

2   Bicker, U., Ziegler, A.E. and Hebold, G. 2[2-cyanaziridinyl-(1)]-2-[2-carbamoylaziridinyl-(1)]propane, BM 12531: a new substance with immune stimulating action. IRCS Med. Sci. 5, 299, 1976.

3   Boerner, D., Bicker, U., Ziegler, A.E., Stosick, U. and Peters, H.S. Influence of BM 12531 (azimexon) on the lymphocyte transformation and the percentage of active T lymphocytes in vivo and in vitro in man. Cancer Immunol. Immunother 6, 237-242, 1979.

4   Bruley-Rosset, M., Florentin, I., Kiger, N., Schulz, J. and Mathé G. Restoration of impaired immune functions of aged animals by chronic bestatin treatment. Immunology 38, 75-83, 1979.

5   Bruley-Rosset, M., Hercend, T., Martinez, J., Rappaport, H. and Mathé G. Prevention of spontaneous tumors of aged mice by immunopharmacological manipulation: study of immune mechanisms. J. Natl. Cancer Inst., 1981 (in press).

6   Florentin, I., Bruley-Rosset, M., Davigny, M. and Mathé G. Comparison of the effect of BCG and a preparation of heat-killed *Pseudomonas aeruginosa* on the immune responses in mice. in The Pharmacology of Immunoregulation (Werner, G.H. and Floc'h, F. eds), pp. 335-351, 1978, Academic Press; New York.

7   Herberman, R.B., Djeu, J.Y., Kay, H.D., Ortaldo, J.R., Riccardi, C., Bonnard, G.D., Holden, H.T., Fagnani, R., Santoni, A. and Pucceti, P. Natural killer cells : characteristics and regulation of activity. Immunol. Rev. 44, 43-70, 1979.

8   Hobbs, J.R. Influence of azimexon in patients with malignant melanoma. Workshop on animal experiments and clinical investigation with azimexon. Mannheim, 9-10 May, 1980.

9   Makinodan, T. and Albright, J.W. Restoration of impaired immune functions in aging animals: effect of mercaptoethanol in enhancing the reduced primary antibody responsiveness in vitro. Mechanisms of Ageing and Development 10, 325-340, 1979.

10 Mathé G. Cancer active immunotherapy. 1976, Springer-Verlag; Heidelberg.

11 Mickshe, M., Kokoschka, E.M., Sagaster, P. and Bicker, U. Phase I study for a new immunostimulating drug, BM 06002, in man. in Immune Modulation and Control of Neoplasia by Adjuvant Therapy. Progress in Cancer Research, Vol. 7, p.403, 1978.

12 Pouillart, P., Palangié T., Huguenin, P., Morin, P., Gautier, H., Baron, A., Mathé G., Lededente, A. and Botto, G. Cancers épidermoïdes bronchiques inopérables. Etude de la signification pronostique de l'état immunitaire et résultats d'un essai d'immunorestauration par le BCG. Nouv. Presse Med. 7, 265-269, 1978.

13 Roumiantzeff, M., Anderson, C.T., Jacquet, P. and Knoker, W.T. New in vivo methods to assay delayed cutaneous hypersensitivity. pp. 297-306 in Transplantation and Clinical Immunology (Touraine, J.L., Traeger, J., Bétuel, H., Brochier, J., Dubernard, J.M., Revillard, J.P. and Triau, R. eds), Vol. X, pp. 297-306, 1979. Excerpta Medica; Amsterdam.

14 Talmadge, J.E., Meyers, K.M., Prieur, D.J. and Starkey, J.R. Role of NK cells in tumour growth and metastasis in beige mice. Nature 284, 622-624, 1980.

15 Terry, W.D. and Rosenberg, S. (eds) Immunotherapy of Cancer: Present Status of Trials in Man. Elsevier/North-Holland, Amsterdam (in press).

16 Touraine, J.L., Hadden, J.W., Touraine, F., Hadden, E.M., Estensen, R and Good, R.A. Phorbol myristate acetate : a mitogen selective for a T lymphocyte subpopulation. J. Exp. Med. 145, 460-465 1977.

CHAPTER 9

Immunopharmacology of DTC in mice and men

Gérard Renoux, Micheline Renoux, Yvon Lebranchu and Pierre Bardos

Laboratoire d'Immunologie, Faculté de Médecine, Tours (France)

SUMMARY

An augmenting agent must be of known pharmacological activity and toxicity, and its ability, on definite cell populations, to restore immunocompetence should be familiar.

Available data indicate that sodium diethyldithiocarbamate, DTC, fulfills most of the requirements. The purified preparation has a very low acute or chronic toxicity in animals. Phase I–II studies in man show that DTC, at immunostimulant doses, has no adverse effects on biochemical and hematological parameters, and no non-immunologic clinical signs.

Repeated, as well as unique, administration of DTC evokes enhanced immune responses, in contrast with most so-called immuno-potentiators. DTC is active on the T-cell lineage, without direct effects on B cells or polyclonal activity. The agent increases all of the following: the percentage of Lyt-1^+ cells, responses to T-cell mitogens or alloantigens, delayed-type hypersensitivities, and the production of antibodies of the IgG class. DTC has no direct effect in vitro. Its influence is mediated through the production, even in congenitally athymic mice, of serum factors inducing T-cell maturation, and it is active across the species barrier. DTC can also enhance NK reactivity. In man, DTC increases the responses to T-cell mitogens, even in cancer patients who have been submitted to surgery. Thus, DTC should be useful in the treatment of diseases or syndromes associated with modified T-cell functions.

9.1. INTRODUCTION

The clinical need for agents to modify the immune response of patients with impaired or depressed resistance has led to the development of a variety of biological and chemical substances with immunomodulatory activities. However, the empirical utilization of agents of half-proven activity, and perhaps built on unwisely chosen models, such as infection-induced macrophage proliferation, has resulted in misunderstandings of the effectiveness of immunotherapy. Learning from the pioneers' works and the increased knowledge today of basic and clinical immunology should serve to avoid some of the now obvious pitfalls in the study of new agents.

In general, an agent augmenting biological responses should comply with the following: no carcinogenicity or tumor-enhancing influence; no antigenic and sensitizing properties; known pharmacological and toxic effects; known effects on the various populations and subsets of immunocompetent cells.

These requirements are needed to reasonably eliminate most of the errors that have been made in the recent past, on the indications and use of immuno-potentiators. Clinical assays should refer not only to survival rate but also to immunoenhancement and its relationship with clinical improvement, prior to assigning a value to a treatment. Unlike chemotherapeutic agents, immuno-potentiators are intended to act on the host to modify his defence mechanisms.

Both experimental knowledge and its clinical confirmation are of paramount importance. For example, an increased number of suppressor cells could favorably modify the lupus-like disease of NZB/W mice, while a similar drug-induced increase in suppressor cells may be deleterious in some cancer cases. Clearly, the deliberate or inadvertent omission of these rules led to the production of conflicting data which was difficult to interpret for further progress.

In light of this we present the unique properties of DTC as an augmenting agent.

9.2. PHARMACOLOGY

9.2.1. Chemistry, toxicology and pharmacology

Sodium diethyldithiocarbamate, DTC, mol.wt 171 (Fig. 9.1) is obtained by reacting diethylamine with carbon disulphide in the presence of sodium hydroxide. It is readily soluble in water, buffers or culture media.

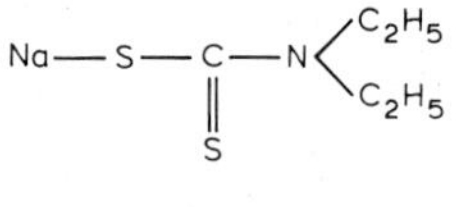

Fig.9.1. The formula of sodium diethyldithiocarbamate. DTC.

The pharmacology and toxicology of DTC has been extensively studied, and recently reviewed [10,40].

DTC is a chelating agent. Administration to animals of large doses (above 200 mg kg^{-1}) produces the following effects:

inhibition of the dopamine-β-hydroxylase, and concomitant depression in brain norepinephrine levels;

potentiation of barbital sleep;

retrograde amnesia of trained passive avoidance;

a dose of 680 mg kg^{-1} produces cerebral seizure activity.

These effects of DTC on catecholamine levels, and liver microsomal enzymes are interesting, as it is almost a rule in pharmacological studies that the effect of low doses contrasts with the activity of high doses.

DTC was also found, at high doses, to temporarily modify blood sugar levels, with no accompanying changes in the histology of adrenals, liver, pituitary and pancreatic islet cells. However, DTC prevents the development of chemically induced diabetes.

The acute toxicity of DTC is low, at an LD$_{50}$ of 1–1.5g kg^{-1}, by the intraperitoneal route. Chronic injections produce the first symptoms (convulsions) at doses higher than 0.5 g per kg/day when prolonged for months.

DTC, as a chelating agent, is used in the treatment of metal poisoning. At daily doses of 30 – 50 mg kg^{-1} body weight, the agent did not produce toxic or untoward side effects, provided sedatives and psychopharmacologic drugs were not concomitantly administered [17,40].

9.2.2. Absence of carcinogenicity. Anti-cancer effects. Radio-protective properties

A recent NCI report [14] relates a bioassay of DTC conducted by administering the chemical in feed for 104–109 weeks to F 344 rats and (B6C3) F$_1$ mice. Briefly, the survival times of the rats and mice were not affected, and no clinical signs could be related to the administration of the drug. The data show (Cox test at $P = 0.025$) that the high dose (about 140 mg per day) prolongs the survival of female mice.

Sufficient numbers of dosed and control animals of each species and sex were at risk for the development of late-appearing tumors. No tumors occurred in the rats or mice at incidences that were significantly higher in the dosed groups compared to the control groups. In addition, the incidence of some spontaneous tumors was lower in the dosed groups than in the corresponding control groups. It is concluded that under the condition of this bioassay, DTC was not carcinogenic for F 344 or B6C3 F$_1$ mice of either sex.

DTC exerts a protective effect against a variety of chemically induced malignant tumors, such as tumors resulting from exposure to polycyclic hydrocarbons [41]; dimethylhydrazine-induced colonic cancer [5,42,43], which effect contrasts with the enhancing effect of C. parvum [3]; liver hepatoma due to azodyes[6].

DTC has been found to be a free radical scavenger [13], protecting rats against the carcinogenic effects of dimethylnitrosamine, probably by preventing DNA strand breaks, or through the effects of DTC on liver enzymes to modify the metabolic pathways of carcinogens [1,37].

In addition, administration of DTC inhibits in rats the nephrotoxicity of, reduces the weight loss from and the gastro-intestinal toxicity of *cis*-platinum [2].

The doses employed in these studies (200–540 mg kg^{-1}) were higher than the doses (0.5–25 mg kg^{-1}) tested for activity on the immune system. The data are, thus, good evidence for the potential safe use of DTC in the clinics.

The beneficial influences of DTC against the lethal effects of ionizing radiation have been reviewed by Strömme and Eldjarn [39]. DTC was found to be a protective agent better than cysteamine, dimethyldithiocarbamate or tetraethylthiuram disulfide.

9.2.2.1. Antibacterial or anti-parasitic activities

DTC has been found to possess in vivo activity against *Mycobacteria, Staphylococci, Enterobacteria, Brucella, Mycoplasma* and spirochetes [4,7,8,11,18]. Such activity might be of interest either against the infections frequently associated with immunodeficiencies and cancers, or in combined antibiotics and immunostimulant therapy of infectious diseases.

9.2.3. Toxico-pharmacology of purified DTC in animals

Commercially available DTC is contaminated with 8 – 10% of a toxic reddish impurity. Purified and lyophilized DTC preparation (Institut Mérieux) is essentially devoid of toxicity and side effects for use as an immunopotentiator.

Acute toxicity by the intravenous route is above 1 g kg^{-1}.

Chronic iv administration of 10 – 100 mg kg^{-1}, 6 days a week for 4 weeks, in beagle dogs and rabbits of either sex, does not evidence toxic effects, changes in eye, heart and blood vessel clinical examination, and hematological or biochemical tests. As complete an examination as possible of the histopathology was identical to that of untreated controls. Similar findings, that is the absence of abnormalities, are observed in 4-month toxicity and pharmacology tests with 20 or 100 mg per kg per day, by the oral route.

Current studies on monkeys (Institut Mérieux) also show similar data, and the absence of any heart or brain lesions detectable by electrographic recording.

9.2.3.1. Anabolic effect of DTC

At the doses tested for augmenting activities, 0.5 – 25 mg kg^{-1}, DTC does not modify the weight of treated animals in comparison with saline-treated controls. In sharp contrast, a treatment with DTC suppresses the wasting disease induced in mice by injecting 2 mg of PMF, a phenol fraction from *Brucella melitensis* [22]. A single administration of as low as 2.5 mg kg^{-1} DTC is sufficient to prevent emaciation (Fig.9.2). Furthermore, DTC-treated mice at the time of PMF injection, exhibited 25 days later a weight increase of 4 – 5 g per animal above that of saline-treated controls. The unique anabolic effect of DTC on animals stressed by a toxic bacterial fraction, might be of interest for the potential use of the agent in cancer patients.

9.2.3.2. Influences of DTC on mouse spleen weight or lymphocyte numbers

In contrast with immunoadjuvants of bacterial origin, DTC does not modify the

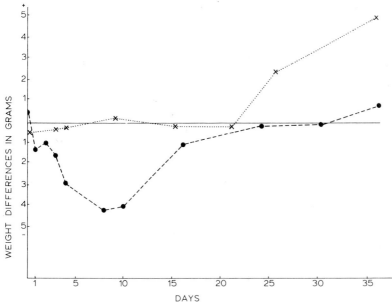

Fig. 9.2. Anabolic effect of DTC on mice emaciated by administering a *Brucella melitensis* cell wall fraction. Heavy line; control, untreated 20 g female mice: •– – –•; *B. melitensis* endotoxin effect (2.5 g/mouse): X– – – –X one DTC treatment, 12 h after endotoxin.

spleen weight in treated mice. If it had any effect, DTC, administered at the time of immunization, would only induce splenocontraction, in comparison with control animals immunized with sheep red blood cells (SRBC) [20,22]. The treatments with DTC leave unchanged the total number of nucleated spleen cells. However, such treatments result in an increased percentage of live cells, in comparison with controls [22]. The cell-protective effect of DTC might have a relationship with its radio-protective efficacy.

The data [20,22,23] show that the immunostimulation afforded by DTC is not associated with a random proliferation of all cells involved in the immune system.

9.2.4. Toxico-pharmacology of purified DTC in man.

All above findings, together with the immunological findings, were found promising enough to permit Phase I–II trials of the purified and lyophilized DTC (Institut Mérieux).

Informed consent was obtained from 29 volunteers: 16 male patients, 38 – 73 years of age, affected with chronic bronchitis, and 13 cancer patients of either sex, 48 – 83 years old.

The data [33,35] can be summarized simply as follows. The slow intravenous administration of $0.5 - 5$ mg kg^{-1} body weight of DTC was devoid of toxicity, and untoward effects, or changes in clinical, hematological, and biochemical parameters. Similar results were obtained on 12 additional chronic bronchitis patients, and are also observed in a current double-blind study on the effects of a weekly repeated treatment with 5 mg kg^{-1} DTC where, at present, no clinical differences are observed among patients.

Immunostimulant doses of purified DTC are devoid of toxicity, adverse effects on brain activity, and synergistic activity with sedatives and anesthetics. DTC should be slowly administered, over more than 10 min, if administered by the intravenous route. Current studies (Lemarie) indicate that oral, aerosol or intrathecal administration of DTC can be as safe and as active as intravenous injection.

9.3 IMMUNOLOGIC ACTIVITIES OF DTC IN MICE

Although we are well aware of the fact that genetic and epigenetic factors can modify the immunoenhancing efficacy of an agent [24], this report will deal mostly with the influence of a 25 mg kg^{-1} dose of DTC on immune responses of female C3H/He (C3) mice.

DTC was found inactive when assayed in vitro and devoid of polyclonal activity [20,22,26,33].

9.3.1. Influence of DTC on T-dependent cell responses

The administration of DTC increases proliferative responses to the T-cell mitogens PHA and Con A, alloantigens in one-way mixed lymphocyte cultures (MLC), specific antibody responses to immunization with SRBC, and delayed-type hypersensitivities.

9.3.1.1. DTC increases the T-cell mitogen-induced lymphoproliferative responses

Splenic cell suspension adjusted to 5×10^6 viable cells per ml was mixed with an equal volume of medium containing either 2 µg kg^{-1} PHA (Wellcome, Beckenham, England), 4 µg ml^{-1} Con A (Calbiochem-Behring, Paris, France) 10 µg ml^{-1} PWM (IBF, Clichy, France) in RPMI-1640 containing 5% inactivated fetal calf serum, FCS (Flow), 2 mM glutamine, 100 U ml^{-1} penicillin, and 100 µg ml^{-1} streptomycin. Then, 0.2 ml of the mixtures containing 0.5×10^6 cells were added to wells of sterile flat-bottom microplates (No. 3040, Falcon Div. Becton-Dickinson, Oxnard, Calif.). Triplicate cultures were incubated for 48 h, at which time 0.5 µCi[3H]thymidine (spec. act. 2 Ci mol^{-1}, CEA, France) was added to each culture. After an additional 18h, the cultures were harvested onto glass-fibre filters and [^{3}H]thymidine incorporation determined by liquid scintillation spectrometry.

As shown in Fig. 9.3, administration of 25 mg kg^{-1} DTC to female C3 mice enhances, when tested 4 days later, the lymphoproliferation induced by Con A, and even more, the PHA-induced response, but left unchanged the proliferative response evoked by PWM.

9.3.1.2. DTC increases the lymphoproliferation induced by alloantigens

C3 (H-2^k) spleen cells were cultured in supplemented RPMI, as above, in 20 ml vol. at a concentration of 1×10^6 cells/ml. Stimulating B6 (H-2^b) spleen cells (mitomycin-treated) were added at a 2×10^6 cells ml^{-1} concentration (1:2 ratio).

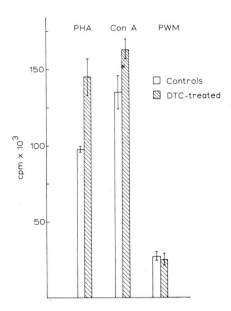

Fig. 9.3. Influence of DTC on the proliferative response to mitogens of C3H/He spleen cells. Tests were performed (see text) 4 days after subcutaneous administration of 25 mg kg[-1] DTC to 16–17 week-old female C3H/He mice.

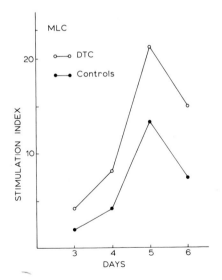

Fig. 9.4. Influence of DTC on the proliferative response to alloantigens of C3H/He spleen cells. Tests were performed (see text for technique) on days 3–6 after subcutaneous administration of 25 mg kg[-1] DTC to 11–12 week-old female C3H/He mice.

Proliferation was evaluated on days 3 to 6 by measuring [^{3}H]thymidine uptake. Triplicate 200-µl aliquots were removed and cultured in microtiter plates with 1 µCi [^{3}H]thymidine for 8–12 h. Samples were harvested onto glass-fibre filters and labelled thymidine incorporation was determined as above.

Fig. 9.4. summarizes the findings. A treatment of female C3 mice with 25 mg kg^{-1} DTC markedly increased, above that of saline-treated controls, the proliferative response of their splenocytes to mitomycin-treated, H-2 incompatible, stimulating cells at each day of assay.

9.3.1.3. DTC increases the specific antibody responses to SRBC

The influence of 25 mg kg^{-1} DTC on the antibody responses to immunization with SRBC was evaluated by a limited in gel hemolysis technique, already described [19,20]. DTC was sc administered simultaneously with iv immunization with 1×10^8 SRBC, and direct (IgM) and indirect (IgG) antibody plaque-forming spleen cells (PFC) were counted 3 – 5 days later. Data were expressed as mean ± S.E.M. of IgM-, or IgG-PFC 10^{-6} viable splenocytes.

Figs. 9.5. and 9.6. show that both the IgM, and the IgG α-SRBC responses were evidently augmented, above that of saline-treated controls, in DTC-treated mice, by a 2.4-fold and a 2.7-fold increase, respectively, at day 4.

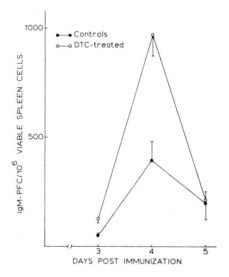

Fig. 9.5. Influence of DTC on α-SRBC IgM-PFC response of female C3H/He spleen cells. Direct (IgM)-PFC were evaluated on days 3–5 after iv immunization with 1×10^8 SRBC and simultaneous sc treatment with 25 mg kg^{-1} DTC.

9.3.1.4. Development of DTH and its persistence in DTC-treated mice

A single treatment with DTC, at the time of immunization, elicits in mice immunized with SRBC higher and longer sustained levels of delayed-type hypersensitivity (DTC) than in controls [22].

Female C3 mice were sensitized with 10^8 SRBC intravenously injected at day 0,

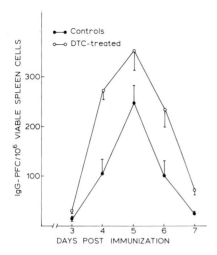

Fig. 9.6.   Influence of DTC on α-SRBC IgG-SRBC response of female C3H/He spleen cells. Indirect (IgG)-PFC were evaluated on days 3–5 after iv immunization with 1×10^8 SRBC and simultaneous sc treatment with 25 mg kg^{-1} DTC.

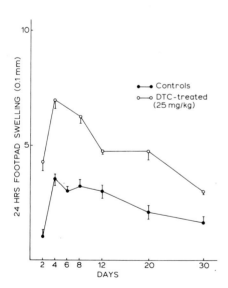

Fig. 9.7.   Influence of DTC on delayed-type hypersensitivity induced by an excess of SRBC. Development and decay in saline-treated mice and in mice treated with 25 mg kg^{-1} DTC at the time of intravenous immunization with 10^8 SRBC. Mice treated with 2.5 mg kg^{-1} DTC are not represented, as the findings were very similar to those of the controls. Means ± SEM of 10 mice per time point.

and simultaneously treated with DTC. According to Lagrange et al. [12], whose technique was followed to measure the increase in footpad thickness, this dose of SRBC fails to sensitize normal untreated mice.

Fig. 9.7. shows that animals treated with 25 mg kg^{-1} DTC display a sharp early peak of DTC response, starting at day 2, which was sustained throughout the time of observation. In contrast, the same dose was unable to modify significantly above controls the DTC response, when sensitization was induced by a suboptimal dose of antigen, 1×10^5 SRBC. In such circumstances, a treatment with 2.5 mg kg^{-1} DTC induced a DTH response that was augmented earlier, reached a higher peak and persisted longer than in untreated controls (Fig. 9.8.). This dose (2.5 mg kg^{-1}) was found ineffective in mice sensitized with 10^8 SRBC.

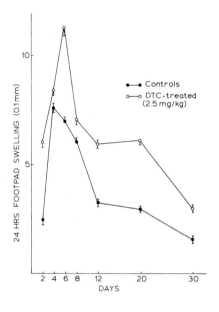

Fig. 9.8. Influence of DTC on DTH induced by a suboptimal dose of SRBC. Development and decay in saline-treated mice and in mice treated with 2.5 mg kg^{-1} DTC at the time of intravenous immunization with 10^5 SRBC. Mice treated with 25 mg kg^{-1} are not represented, as their responses were not significantly differing from those of controls. Means ± SEM of 10 mice per time point.

The data indicate that DTC affects the macrophage- and T-cell-induced delayed-type hypersensitivity response to SRBC. It is of interest for further studies, and correlation with clinical assay, to lay stress on the finding that a high dose of DTC, 25 mg kg^{-1}, enhances response when an excess of antigen is present, whereas a low dose of the agent, 2.5 mg kg^{-1}, increases an already positive DTH response. Interesting also is the finding that DTC can impair the immediate antibody-mediated hypersensitivity to DNP and enhance the delayed hypersensitivity to BGG in guinea pigs immunized with BGG-DNP[15].

Thus, a single injection of DTC to female C3 mice increases either the proliferative responses to T-cell mitogens and alloantigens, the antibody responses against a complex antigen, SRBC, or delayed-type-hypersensitivities. These effects were not accompanied with an influence of DTC on the B-cell mitogen (at least, for mice) PWM. The results correlate with previous findings evidencing the efficacy of DTC to recruit Thy-1$^+$ cells from precommitted precursor spleen cells in *nu/nu* mice, without apparent changes in the number of B(CR$^+$) cells [20,22,29,31,33].

Current studies are in progress to determine whether the helper effect of DTC is associated with modifications in the relative percentages of T-cell subsets, and/or modifications of the relative amounts of cell-surface antigens, as markers of differences in the expression of the products of the MHC complex.

9.3.2. Influence of DTC on T-cell surface antigens

Administration of DTC to C3 mice was found to increase the percentage of Thy-1$^+$ spleen cells [26,33]. To determine the influence of DTC on T-cell subsets, the percentage of Lyt$^+$ subsets was evaluated in spleen cells of C3 mice, 4 days after a treatment with 25 mg kg^{-1} DTC, by a two-step cytotoxic assay using monoclonal antibodies and complement.

Table 9.I. shows the results of one such experiment. DTC increased the number of Lyt-1$^+$ spleen cells significantly above that of saline-treated controls ($P<0.01$), at the expense of the Lyt-1,2,3$^+$ set, which decreased to half the value for untreated controls. A similar increase in the number of Lyt-1$^+$ cells was also found in lymph node cells of DTC-treated mice (data not shown).

Table 9.I.

Influence of 25 mg kg^{-1} DTC on spleen Lyt subsets

Treatment	Percent of:		
	Lyt-1$^+$	Lyt-2.3$^+$	Lyt-1.2.3$^+$
Saline	9.0	5.0	10.0
DTC	16.5	3.0	5.0

Enumeration of the Lyt subsets was performed by the technique of Reske-Kunz et al. [36], using monoclonal α-Lyt-1.1 (No. FPA 172) and α-Lyt-2.1 (No. FPA 066, NEN, Boston) antibodies, both at the 1:750 dilution, low-tox M rabbit complement (Cedarlane) at the 1:10 dilution. Specific lysis was evaluated by the trypan blue exclusion test. Percentage specific lysis was calculated by the formula 100 × ($a−b$) (100−b), where a and b represent the percentage lysis obtained in the presence of specific antibody and normal mouse serum, respectively. There were four mice per group.

9.3.3. DTC as a trigger of hormone-like factors

9.3.3.1. Effect on mice.
DTC is inactive in in vitro tests, in contrast with levamisole, the in vitro activity of

which was found to be associated to the cholinergic-like effects of its imidazole moiety [9,20].

DTC induces the in vivo acquisition of specific T-cell markers by precommitted, and undifferentiated, precursor spleen cells in congenitally thymus-devoid mice and concomitantly, functional immune activation [21,23,30,32,34]. Table 9.II. represents a further experiment performed with the semi-automated microcytotoxicity assay [28] and monoclonal α-Thy-1 antibody. The results confirm previous data, illustrate the T-cell recruiting ability of DTC without influence on the total number of B cells, and suggest a dose-response effect.

Table 9.II.

In vivo generation of T cells in *nu/nu* mice. 4 days after a treatment with DTC

Treatment (mg kg^{-1})	Percent of induced cells Thy-1^{+a}	Percent of CR$^+$ spleen cells[b]
Saline[d]	0	33 – 38
DTC, 2.5	17 – 19[c]	24 – 29
DTC, 25	20 – 29	16 – 32

[a]Nett increase above background (2–6 Thy-$^+$ cells). [b]Total number of B(CR$^+$) cells, enumerated by a modification of the Bianco et al. test as developed by Scheid et al. [38]. [c]Minimum and maximum percent evaluated. [d]Four – 6 mice per group.

The serum of DTC-treated *nu/nu* mice transfers, like the serum of treated thymus-bearing mice, in vivo activities and allows precursor spleen cells of *nu/nu* mice to differentiate in vitro into Thy-1$^+$ cells. As shown in Table 9.III., 0.01 ml of serum, sampled on *nu/nu* mice 4 days after a treatment with 25 mg kg^{-1} DTC, induced the appearance of about 20% Thy-1$^+$ cells in a 3.5 h induction assay on

Table 9.III.

In vitro generation of T cells by the serum of *nu/nu* mice treated with DTC

Inducer 0.01 ml	Percent of Thy-1$^+$ induced[a]	Percent of CR$^+$ spleen cells[b]
RPMI-1640 medium	0 – 5[c]	24 – 32
nu/nu mouse serum	0 – 3	18 – 28
Serum from DTC-treated *nu/nu* mice	20 – 24	19 – 26

nu/nu Mice (C57 background) were treated with 25 mg kg^{-1} DTC, 4 days prior to sampling. For captions, see Table 9.II.

nu/nu spleen cells, whereas even a 18 h incubation was unable to modify the percentage of B(CR$^+$) cells.

At present, DTC (and DTC-induced serum factor) is the only known agent to induce in thymus-less mice the in vivo acquisition of specific T-cell markers by undifferentiated precursor lymphoid cells, following a single administration of the agent.

9.3.3.2. Activity across species barriers of the DTC-induced serum factor

Mouse serum was obtained 24 h after a sc injection of 25 mg kg^{-1} of DTC to female BALB/c mice. Its ability to induce HTLA$^+$ cells or CR$^+$ cells was tested on a mixture of peripheral blood lymphocytes deprived of mature T cells by repeated depletion of E rosettes on a density gradient. After a 4 h incubation at 37°C in a humidified atmosphere of 5 % CO$_2$ in the presence of mouse serum, the cells with surface T-lymphocyte differentiation antigens (HTLA$^+$ cells) were identified in a microcytotoxicity assay, and CR$^+$B cells were counted, after 6 or 18 h of incubation [26].

The populations studied include 54–57% CR$^+$ cells, before and after 18 h in vitro incubation, and show the absence of effect on the B-cell lineage of DTC-treated mouse serum.

Between 2 and 6% of cells with the HTLA phenotype remain after elimination of the E-rosette forming cells. The data presented in Table 9.IV show that a 4-h incubation of E$^-$ human lymphocytes with as low as 10 µl of serum of DTC-treated BALB/c mice was sufficient to convert an additional 7 – 12% HTLA$^-$ cells into HTLA$^+$ cells, at a level comparable to the effect of calf thymus extract.

Table 9.IV.

In vitro generation of HTLA$^+$ cells from human E$^-$ cells by serum from DTC-treated mice

Treatment	% nett increase of HTLA+		
	(1)	(2)	(3)
10 µl SF	7.8	12.2	12.5
20 µl SF	17.5	15.0	13.0
50 µl F3V	13.2	11.6	10.4
20 µl NMS	0	2.3	4.4

NMS, normal mouse serum; F3V, calf-thymus extract, 1 mg ml^{-1} proteins; SF, DTC-treated BALB/c mouse serum. Figures in parentheses indicate three separate experiments.

The serum of DTC-treated mice is also capable of increasing functional activities of human peripheral blood lymphocytes, as measured by the enhancement of Con A-induced proliferation. In addition, blast cells induced by Con A or by the serum of DTC-treated mice suppressed equally the proliferative response in MLC, in contrast to the blasts induced by calf thymus extract, which did not display a significant suppressor activity [26].

In conclusion, DTC appears to promote or to stimulate the in vivo synthesis of a potent inducer of prothymocyte maturation and acquisition of functional activities. This inducer is active across species barriers.

9.3.4. Influences of DTC on NK and ADCC of female C3H/He mice

Natural killer activity and antibody-dependent cell-mediated cytotoxicity (ADCC), were measured in a 4-h, ^{51}Cr-release assay. The YAC-1 subline of YAC lymphoma cells, induced by Moloney murine leukemia virus in strain A mice was maintained in vitro in RPMI-1640 medium supplemented with 10% heat-inactivated FCS, 100 U ml^{-1} penicillin, 50 μg ml^{-1} streptomycin and 0.05 mM 2-mercaptoethanol. Chicken erythrocytes (CRBC) were obtained from young fowl, using heparin as anti-coagulant. After three washes in sterile saline, CRBC suspensions were adjusted to 5 × 10^6 cells ml^{-1}, coated with heat-inactivated anti-CRBC (Cappel, Cochranville, PA) at 1:1500 dilution, and thoroughly washed in Hank's balanced-salt solution.

Target cells, YAC cells for NK activity, sensitized CRBC for ADCC activity, were labelled with 100 μCi ^{51}Cr per 1.5 × 10^6 cells for 60 min at 37°C. Cytotoxicities were measured in triplicate samples at target to effector ratios (E/T) of 100:1 – 6:1 with 1.0 – 1.25 × 10^4 target cells and evaluated by the formula: 100 × (mean cpm experimental — mean cpm spontaneous release)/(mean cpm maximum release — mean cpm spontaneous release).

Spontaneous release was determined by incubating target cells in medium alone; maximum release was determined by detergent lysis.

Fig. 9.9 and 9.10 summarize the data from 4 – 6 mice per test. As shown in Fig. 9.9, a treatment with 25 mg kg^{-1} DTC, 4 days before the test, significantly ($P < 0.01$) increases the NK activity of female C3 mice at E/T ratios from 1:25 to 1:100, whereas this treatment is unable to modify ADCC to CRBC (Fig. 9.10). The data are to be confirmed by other experiments, including variable time- and dose-schedules of treatment, and other mouse strains of different genetic level of NK activity. If confirmed, the specific stimulating effect of DTC on NK reactivity and its inability to trigger an increased ADCC on erythrocytes, will provide a means to further delineate the cell subsets active in the resistance to tumors.

9.3.5. Influence of DTC on mice immunosuppressed by chemotherapeutic agents

In view of its potential use in cancer therapy, DTC was chronically administered (25 mg kg^{-1} 3-times a week for 4 weeks) to BALB/c mice treated for 4 weeks with therapeutic-like doses of cyclophosphamide (CY), azathioprine (AZA) or cortisone acetate HC [25].

Immune responses were evaluated by mitogen-induced lymphocyte proliferation and by in vivo primary antibody responses to SRBC. Half the number of mice were killed for lymphoproliferative assays, and the other half were immunized with 10^8 SRBC, 4 days after the end of treatment to minimize the role of residual drug activity or of stress on lymphocyte responsiveness. The administration of DTC

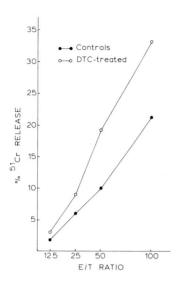

Fig. 9.9.   Influence of DTC on the NK reactivity of C3H/He spleen cells. 12-week-old female C3H/He mice were treated with 25 mg kg⁻¹ DTC, 4 days prior to killing and test. For technique see text. Means of 4 mice per group.

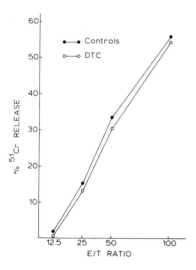

Fig. 9.10.   Influence of DTC on the antibody-dependent cell-mediated cytotoxicity (ADCC) to chicken erythrocytes of C3H/He spleen cells. 12-week-old female C3H/He mice were treated with 25 mg kg⁻¹ DTC, 4 days prior to killing and test. For technique see text. Means of 4 mice per group.

alone, even for 1 month, stimulated the host to increased T-cell associated responses.

Chronic treatments with the chemotherapeutic agents impaired, or inhibited, mitogen-induced lymphoproliferations and antibody responses. DTC, administered simultaneously with AZA or HC, increased these responses above that of untreated controls, at levels comparable to those of mice treated with DTC alone, and partially restored the responses abrogated by CY. The results are encouraging as they raise the possibility of developing a rational chemoimmunotherapy using DTC in association with a compatible cytoreductive drug.

9.4. EFFECTS OF DTC ON IMMUNE PARAMETERS IN MAN

The effects of DTC were evaluated on the informed-consent volunteers of the Phase I–II preliminary studies, by the following tests: serum levels of IgA, IgG and IgM, total hemolytic complement (CH50), and C4 and C3; T cells (E rosettes) and B cells (Ig-bearing cells, by immunofluorescence); response to PHA and Con A after 72 h of culture, and addition of 5 μCi [^{3}H]thymidine per ml for the last 18 h of incubation.

Tests were performed before administering DTC (day 0) and at days +1, +2 and +7 after each injection.

In an initial series of assays, low doses of DTC (0.5– 2.2 mg kg^{-1} per iv injection) were administered to cancer patients, prior to surgery. In all cases but one (a 70-year-old woman severely affected by recurrent breast cancer and extensive radio-dermitis on the thorax), the responses to T-cell mitogens were restored to normal levels, or even above. Thus, low doses of DTC prevent the well-known immunodepression associated with surgery and anesthesia, in patients whose immune responses are already altered by cancer [35].

A second series was made up of male patients affected with chronic pulmonary infections. They were treated with 5 mg kg^{-1} DTC. Results have been published elsewhere [33,35], but Table 9.V. summarizes the findings extended to 28 patients.

A single administration of DTC increased to normal values the responses of PHA or Con A that were impaired prior to treatment (day 0). The percentage of T cells returned to normal values, either when the figure was abnormally high or low at day 0 before treatment.

The following tests were not affected by the treatment: percent of B (sIg$^+$) cells, levels of IgA, IgG, IgM, or complement activity in the serum. The percent of autologous rosette-forming cells was lowered ($\bar{m}$ 15.35) in all patients, and not affected by the treatment with DTC.

In man, as in animals, DTC was not a polyclonal activator. The mean values of background responses (cpm $\pm$ SE in the absence of mitogens) were : 638 $\pm$ 504 at day 0, 737 $\pm$ 541 at day +1, 482 $\pm$ 343 at day +2, and 554 $\pm$ 400 at day +7.

These preliminary results confirm in man the unique, and specific influence of DTC to regulate the activities of the T-cell lineage, without apparent, direct effect on B cells.

9.5. DISCUSSION

The use of the immunomodifying properties of a number of agents for

Table 9.V.

A summary of the influence of 5 mg kg^{-1} DTC on the responses of peripheral blood lymphocytes of chronic bronchitis patients

Test	Day of testing			
	0	+ 1	+ 2	+ 7
E rosettes (28)	64.5	64.25	64.25	61.35
Low E rosettes (15)	54.12	53.75	60.75	60.12
High E rosettes (13)	73.62	72.12	68.12	63.12*
PHA (28)	28701	38897	30910	47743*
Con A (28)	21392	21521	25320	32623*

These figures were compared to 202 normal healthy controls for E rosettes (65 ± 5), PHA (38 635 ± 8 635) and Con A (41 415 ± 8 935), and 53 healthy controls for autologous rosette-forming cells (24 ± 2.9). In the table, figures in parentheses indicate the number of patients. The 28 data (first line) on percent of T cells were analyzed by subdividing the group into two parts : 15 patients with T-cell (E rosettes) percentage below, and 13 patients with E rosettes above that of normal controls. *Significant at $P<0.01$.

immunotherapy has pushed back the known limitations of conventional therapies against cancers. However, their empirical utilization without sufficient knowledge of their modes of action, associated with uncontrolled clinical assays, has led to disappointment about the potential usefulness of immunotherapy. "It is clear that immunotherapy as presently practised has fallen far short of the hopes initially invested in it..." [16]. We should emphasize "*as presently practised*". Indeed, advances in immunopharmacology and clinical immunology, and the hope that a closer discourse between clinicians and fundamentalists will be established, should provide a new basis to evaluate the true role of immunology in cancers.

Our aim is to obtain enough straightforward data to enable the clinician to make his own decision and choice of application in known, selected cases.

Although analysis is far from complete, the findings suggest a unique influence of DTC on the immune system.

DTC in its purified form, is a non-toxic agent devoid of untoward pharmacological effects, at least at the doses effective on immunity.

The administration of DTC induces the maturation (recruitment?) of T cells from undifferentiated precursor cells.

DTC increases the Lyt-1$^+$ set which, in turn, induces (i) other T cells to generate enhanced levels of cytotoxic activities, (ii) macrophages and monocytes to participate in delayed-type-hypersensitivity, (iii) B cells to secrete antibodies of the IgG class and, probably, (iv) resting T cells to develop suppressive activities. DTC augments the NK reactivity of C3 mice. DTC has no direct influence on B cells, nor polyclonal activities, or in vitro enhancing effects.

The influence of DTC is due to the increased synthesis, even in congenitally athymic mice, of hormone-like factors active on T-cell lineage. This synthesis appears to be under the control of the brain neocortex [27,29,34].

In contrast with most of the so-called immunopotentiators, responses above that of untreated controls are obtained after chronic administration of DTC, as well as after a single treatment.

One could, therefore, predict the efficacy of DTC in syndromes or diseases known to be associated with impaired, or inhibited, T-cell responses. It can comprise not only cancers, but also some autoimmune diseases.

Preliminary studies in man conform with these views. Administration of DTC is not followed by changes in the hematological and biochemical parameters, nor by toxic effects. Such a treatment increases for about one week the response of peripheral blood lymphocytes to T-cell mitogens, to such an extent that it prevents in aged cancer patients the immunodepression caused by surgical trauma and restores the impaired responses associated with cancer.

We hope that DTC might prove its usefulness in the preoperative management of cancer patients to obviate the immune impairment provoked by surgery, thus reducing the risk of disseminating micro-metastases. In as much as the immune system contributes to the elimination of neoplasic cells, the use of DTC after radical surgery may prevent metastases or recurrences. DTC could also be the basis for a rational immuno-chemotherapy, and prevent the damage to the immune system induced by radiation therapy.

These hopes are attainable, as DTC satisfies the requirements for a non-toxic agent, devoid of untoward side effects, producing an augmenting effect on the cellular arm of the immune system.

ACKNOWLEDGEMENTS

Supported by a grant-in-aid from the Institut Mérieux. The authors acknowledge Professor L. Gyenes for pertinent advice, Mr J.M. Guillaumin and Mrs C. Gouzien, E. Billand, B. Jean and V. Grodemange for skilful technical assistance.

REFERENCES

1 Abanoni, S.E., Popp, J.A., Chang, S.K., Harrington, G.W., Lotlikar, P.D., Hadjiolov, D., Levitt, M., Rajalakohimi, S. and Sarma, D.R.S. Inhibition of dimethylnitrosamine-induced strand breaks in liver DNA and liver cell necrosis by diethyldithiocarbamate. J. Natl. Cancer Inst. 58, 263, 1977.
2 Borch, R.F. and Pleasant, M.E. Inhibition of cis-platinum nephrotoxicity by diethyldithiocarbamate rescue in rats. Proc. Natl. Acad. Sci. USA 76, 6611, 1979.
3 Cruse, J.P., Lewin, M.R. and Clark, C.G., Corynebacterium parvum enhances colonic cancer in dimethylhydrazine-treated rats. Brit. J. Cancer 37, 639, 1978.
4 Drozdou, N.S. Effect of g-p-dialkylaminophenyl-10 alkylacridine and of dithiocarbamic acid derivatives on spirochetes. Med. Parasitol. Parasitic Diseases (URSS) 11, 92, 1942.
5 Fiala, E.S., Bobotas, G., Kulakis, C., Wattenberg, L.W. and Weisberger, I.H. Effects of disulfuram and related compounds on the metabolism in vivo of the colon carcinogen, 1,2-dimethylhydrazine. Biochem. Pharmacol. 26, 1763, 1977.

6 Fiala, E.S., Fiala, E.A. and Keller, R.W. Activation of γ-glutamyl transferase in rat liver by disulfuram and its effects on the first stage of azo-dye-induced carcinogenesis. Fed. Proc. 36, 349, 1977.

7 Garattini, S. and Leonardi, A. The antituberculous action of chelating substances. Giorn. Ital. Chemother. 2, 18, 1955.

8 Goth, A. and Robinson, F.J. Chemotherapeutic studies on a series of dithiocarbamates and their bismuth derivatives. J. Pharmacol. Exptl. Therap. 93, 430, 1948.

9 Hadden, J.W., Coffey, R.C., Hadden, E.M., Lopez-Corrales, E. and Sunshine, G.H. Effects of levamisole and imidazole on lymphocyte proliferation and cyclic nucleotide levels. Cell. Immunol. 20, 98, 1975.

10 Haley, T.J. Disulfuram (tetraethylperoxidicarbonic diamide): a reappraisal of its toxicity and therapeutic application. Drug Metabol. Rev. 9, 319, 1979.

11 Jeney, E. and Zsolnai, T. Tuberculostatic agents. IV. The chemotherapeutic action of some hydrazine derivatives and organic sulphur compounds on experimental tuberculosis in guinea pigs. Z. Bakt. Parasitenk. I, Origin 167, 254, 1956.

12 Lagrange, P.H., MacKaness, G.B. and Miller, T.E. Influence of dose and route of antigen injection on the immunologic induction of T cells. J. Exp. Med. 139, 528, 1974.

13 Lutz, L.M., Glende, E.A. and Recknagel, R.O. Protection by diethyldithiocarbamate against carbon tetrachloride lethality in rats and against carbon tetrachloride-induced lipid peroxidation in vitro. Biochem. Pharmacol. 22, 1729, 1973.

14 National Cancer Institute. Bioassay of sodium diethyldithiocarbamate for possible carcinogenesis. Tech. Rep. Ser. No. 172, 1979.

15 Neveu, P.J. The effect of thiol moiety of levamisole on both cellular and humoral immunity during the early response to a hapten-carrier complex. Clin. Exp. Immunol. 32, 419, 1978.

16 Nossal, G.J.V. The case history of Mr T.I. Terminal patient or still curable? Immunology Today 1, 5, 1980.

17 Panel on Nickel. Nickel, a report to the committee on medical and biologic effects of environmental pollution, 1957, p. 106, Natl. Acad. Sci.; USA.

18 Renoux, G. and Quatrefages, H. Une nouvelle méthode de différenciation des variétés de *Brucella* : action du diethyldithiocarbamate de soude (DEDTC). Ann. Inst. Pasteur 82, 556, 1952.

19 Renoux, G. and Renoux, M. Modulation of immune reactivity by phenylimidithiazole salts in mice immunized by sheep red blood cells. J. Immunol. 113, 779, 1974.

20 Renoux, G. and Renoux, M. Roles of the imidazole or thiol moiety on the immunostimulant action of levamisole. in Control of Neoplasia by Modulation of the Immune System (Chirigos, M.A. Ed.), p. 67, 1977, Raven Press, New York.

21 Renoux, G. and Renoux, M. Thymus-like activities of sulphur derivatives on T-cell differentiation. J. Exp. Med. 145, 466, 1977 b.

22 Renoux, G. and Renoux, M. Immunopotentiation and anabolism induced by sodium diethyldithiocarbamate. J. Immunopharmacol. 1, 247, 1979.

23 Renoux, G., Renoux, M., Guillaumin, J.M. and Gouzien, C. Differentiation and regulation of lymphocyte populations: evidence for immunopotentiator-induced T cell recruitment. J. Immunopharmacol. 1, 415, 1979.

24 Renoux, G., Renoux, M. and Guillaumin, J.M. Genetic and epigenetic control of levamisole-induced immunostimulation. Internat. J. Immunopharmacol. 1, 43, 1979.

25 Renoux, G. and Renoux M. The effects of sodium diethyldithiocarbamate, azathioprine, cyclophosphamide or hydrocortisone acetate administered alone or in association for 4 weeks on the immune responses of BALB/c mice. Clin. Immunol. Immunopathol. 15, 21, 1980.

26 Renoux, G., Touraine, J.L. and Renoux, M. Induction of differentiation of human null cells into T lymphocytes by the serum of mice treated with sodium diethyldithiocarbamate. J. Immunopharmacol. 2, 49, 1980.

27 Renoux, G., Biziere, K., Renoux, M. and Guillaumin, J.M. Le cortex cérébral règle les réponses immunes des souris. C.R. Acad. Sci. Paris, 710, 2900, 1980.

28 Renoux, G., Gyenes, L., Guillaumin, J.M. and Jean, B. A semi-automated rapid and sensitive microcytotoxicity assay for antibody-mediated cytolysis. J. Immunol. Methods, 36, 71, 1980.

29 Renoux, G., Biziere, K., Renoux, M., Gyenes, L., Degenne, D., Guillaumin, J.M., Bardos, P. and Lebranchu, Y. Effects of the ablation of the left cerebral cortex on T-cell number and cell-mediated responses in the mouse. Internat. J. Immunopharmacol. 2, 156, 1980.

30 Renoux, G., Renoux, M., Gyenes, L. and Guillaumin, J.M. A comparison of the in vivo T-cell recruiting capacity of DTC, serum of DTC-treated mice, and two synthetic thymic hormones. Internat. J. Immunopharmacol. 2, 167, 1980 f.

31 Renoux, G., Renoux, M., Lavandier, M. and Lemarie, E. Clinical pharmacology and immunology of DTC. Internat. J. Immunopharmacol. 2, 168, 1980.

32 Renoux, G. and Renoux, M. Administration of DTC evidences a role of the thymus in the control and regulation of factors inducing thymocyte differentiation in the mouse. Thymus, 2, 139, 1980.

33 Renoux, G. and Renoux, M. Immunologic activity of DTC: a potential for cancer therapy. in Augmenting Agents in Cancer Therapy: Current Status and Future Prospects (Hersh, E.M. and Chirigos, M.A. Eds), pp. 427-440, Raven Press; New York, 1981.

34 Renoux, G., Differentiation of the T-cell lineage by sodium diethyldithiocarbamate (DTC). Influence of the neocortex. in New Trends in Human Immunology and Cancer Immunotherapy (Serrou, B., and Rosenfeld, Cl. Eds), pp. 986-994, Doin-Saunders, 1980.

35 Renoux, G., Renoux, M., Greco, J., Baudoin, J., Lavandier, M. and Lemarie, E. Phase I-II studies of sodium diethyldithiocarbamate (DTC). In New Trends in Human Immunology and Cancer Immunotherapy (Serrou, B. and Rosenfeld, Cl. Eds), pp. 974-985, Doin-Saunders, 1980.

36 Reske-Kunz, A.B., Scheid, M.P. and Boyse, E.A. Disproportion in T-cell subpopulations in immunodeficient mutant nr/nr mice. J. Exp. Med. 149, 228, 1979.

37 Sarma, D.S.R., Rajalakshisni, S. and Hadjiolov, D. Effect of diethyldithiocarbamate (DEDTC) and aminoacetylnitrile (AAN) on the induction of strand breaks in rat liver DNA by chemical carcinogens in vivo. Fed. Proc. 33, 395, 1974.

38 Scheid, M.P., Goldstein, G. and Boyse, E.A. Differentiation of T cells in nude mice. Science 190, 1211, 1975.

39 Stromme, J.H. and Eldjarn, L. Distribution and chemical forms of diethyldithiocarbamate and tetraethylthiuram disulphide (disulfuram) in mice in relation to radioprotection. Biochem. Pharmacol. 15, 287, 1966.

40 Sunderman, P.W. Efficacy of sodium diethyldithiocarbamate (Dithiocarb) in acute nickel carbonyl poisoning. Ann. Clin. Lab. Sci. 9, 1, 1979.

41 Wattenberg, L.W. Inhibition of carcinogenic and toxic effects of polycyclic hydrocarbons by several sulfur-containing compounds. J. Natl. Cancer Inst. 52, 1583, 1974.

42 Wattenberg, L.W. Inhibition of dimethylhydrazine-induced neoplasia of the large intestine by disulfuram. J. Natl. Cancer Inst. 54, 1005, 1975.

43 Wattenberg, L.W. and Fiala, E.S. Inhibition of 1,2-dimethylhydrazine-induced neoplasia of the large intestine in female CP_1 mice by carbon disulfide; brief communication. J. Natl. Cancer Inst. 60, 1515, 1978.

CHAPTER 10

C 1740 (Biostim): an overview of preclinical studies and phase I clinical trial in cancer patients

J.M. Lang[a], C. Giron[a], R. Zalisz[b], C. Marchiani[b], J.P. Buret[b] and F. Oberling[a]

[a] *Service des Maladies du Sang, Hôpital de Hautepierre, Strasbourg (France) and*
[b] *Laboratoires Cassenne et Centre de Recherche Roussel-UCLAF, Paris (France)*

10.1. INTRODUCTION

C 1740 (Biostim) is a glycoproteinic extract from *Klebsiella pneumoniae* serotype 2 (Laboratoires Cassenne and Centre de Recherche Roussel UCLAF, Paris, France). It is a compound with a molecular weight of more than 100 000. Its biochemical analysis has been performed by Professor Montreuil and co-workers at the University of Lille, France, and the following composition has been determined:

Neutral sugars (glucose, galactose, mannose) 50.2%
Glucuronic acid 8.8%
N-Acetyl glucosamine 1.2%
Proteins 26.0%

The main amino acids of the proteinic fraction are aspartic and glutamic acids. The lack of cystein and diaminopimelic acid is a particular feature of C 1740.

After a brief survey of toxicity studies and results of preclinical evaluation of C 1740 relating to its effects on the immune system, we shall describe a very simple short-term clinical assay showing that C 1740 is able to restore and to enhance delayed cutaneous hypersensitivity in cancer patients.

10.2. TOXICITY STUDIES

Acute, subacute and chronic toxicological studies failed to reveal any significant abnormalities in mice, rats, rabbits and monkeys when the compound was given orally. LD_{50} in mice and rats is higher than 1000 mg kg^{-1}. Daily doses up to 100 mg kg^{-1} in rats and 5 mg kg^{-1} in monkeys have been perfectly well tolerated on chronic administration. On the other hand, a daily dose of 5 mg kg^{-1} given intraperitoneally in rats led to 25% mortality after 3 months, with severe local inflammatory lesions and lymphoid hyperplasia. Mesenteric lymph nodes or Peyer patches hyperplasia was never observed with the oral route.

In addition, C 1740 had no teratogenic effects, no effect on fertility or reproduction performance in rats and rabbits, and no mutagen activity.

10.3. PRECLINICAL IN VIVO AND IN VITRO STUDIES : AN OVERVIEW

Immunological studies in animals have been performed in Paris by the groups of C. Griscelli, J.F. Bach, and J. Agneray, as well as by the Centre de Recherche des Laboratoires Cassenne. Data are unpublished yet and since manuscripts are in preparation results will only be summarized here. C 1740 has been shown to protect mice against bacterial infections, to increase blood clearance of living bacteria and carbon particles and to stimulate phagocytosis by both monocytes–macrophages and polymorphonuclear cells. It also behaves as an adjuvant of the humoral immune response to sheep red blood cells in mice and to ovalbumin in guinea pigs. It increases delayed cutaneous hypersensitivity to ovalbumin and dinitrochloroben-zene (DNCB) in guinea pigs. All these effects have been observed with the oral route of administration. Injected into the foot pad of mice C 1740 at a dose range of 5 – 80 μg per mouse increases the weight of the popliteal lymph node. C 1740 is mitogenic for mouse spleen lymphocytes, spleen cells from athymic nude mice (B cells) and for T cells prepared from mouse spleen by filtration on nylon fibers or treatment of spleen cells with anti-Ig serum. However, very recently, Kotani in Japan could not confirm the mitogenic effect of C 1740 on mouse T cells (personal communication), in his hands C 1740 rather would appear as an activator of both B cells and macrophages. Anyhow, the mitogenicity of C 1740 on mouse spleen cells is dose related and polyclonal in nature rather than due to the antigenicity of the compound.

In humans C 1740 has been shown by Griscelli (personal communication) to clearly enhance peripheral blood lymphocyte reactivity to phytohaemagglutinin, Concanavalin A and pokeweed mitogen in vitro, with a maximum of 240% potentiation at C 1740 concentrations of 0.01 – 0.001 μg ml^{-1} added to the medium throughout the culture period. A maximum 170% potentiation was observed when cell suspensions were pre-incubated with the same concentrations of the drug and washed thereafter. There is also evidence from a study by B. Grospierre and C. Griscelli that C 1740 is mitogenic for human peripheral blood lymphocytes (manuscript in preparation). Finally, C 1740 induces chemotaxis of human polymorphonuclear cells in Boyden chambers.

We studied (unpublished data) the effects of C 1740 in vitro on spontaneous rosette formation by peripheral blood lymphocytes (total E rosettes) in a small series of untreated cancer patients. C 1740 was added to the medium throughout the assay to a final concentration of 5 μg ml^{-1}. The same assay was conducted in parallel on the same blood sample without C 1740, as a control. It appeared that C 1740 had no effect on total E rosettes when the percentages were within the normal range. However, when only patients with less than 60% total E rosettes were considered there was an increase of their mean percentage in the presence of C 1740 ($61 \pm 11.6\%$ versus $53.4 \pm 5.5\%$), the difference was only slightly significant ($P = 0.05$ by the Wilcoxons' test) due to the small number of patients ($n = 9$) and to the wide dispersion of individual results. On the other hand, in patients with more than 75% total E rosettes the addition of C 1740 significantly decreased their mean percentage ($71.4\% \pm 7.7$ versus $78.2\% \pm 2.6$, $n = 13$, $P = 0.01$). While it is tempting to view C 1740 as an immunomodulator on the basis of the preceding data, we feel that the small number of patients studied hampered any interpretation.

10.4. PHASE I CLINICAL TRIAL OF C 1740 IN CANCER PATIENTS

Since C 1740 proved to be devoid of any detectable toxicity when given per os and to enhance or stimulate several parameters of the immune response in both animal and man, we decided to set up a phase I short-term clinical trial. The aim of the trial was to test the capacity of C 1740 given per os for a short period of time to restore delayed cutaneous hypersensitivity (DCH) reactions in anergic or hypoergic cancer patients and to enhance DCH in cancer patients with apparently normal skin reactivity. Cancer patients were selected because cancer is frequently associated with defective general parameters of cell-mediated immunity and immune status is of important prognostic significance in these patients. Thus immunorestoration of cancer patients may become in the near future an important part of the therapeutic strategy.

Twenty one consecutive adult patients of both sexes, ranging in age from 16 to 71 years (mean age, 41) entered this open trial. Thirteen, including seven with Hodgkin's disease, were untreated patients tested at the time of pretreatment evaluation. Five were patients relapsing with metastases at a distance from prior treatment. The last three patients had Hodgkin's disease in complete remission. All these patients were unlikely to show spontaneous recovery or increase of skin reactivity to recall antigens during the trial period. They were given no other drug.

Delayed cutaneous hypersensitivity to recall antigens was tested using a plastic disposable multipuncture device (Multitest, Institut Mérieux, Marcy l'Etoile, Charbonnières les Bains 69260, France). This system simultaneously administers eight test materials including a battery of seven standardized glycerinated antigens (tuberculin, tetanus toxoid, diphtheria toxoid, *Streptococcus*, *Candida*, *Trichophyton* and *Proteus* antigens) and a glycerin control. It allows easy quantitation and has provided high reproducibility [4–6], without leading to positive reactions on repeated applications [5]. It thus permits repeated testing in a single individual to recognize significant changes in delayed cutaneous hypersensitivity.

Skin testing was performed 2 days before and immediately after treatment with C 1740. Reactions were evaluated after 48 h by measuring two crossed diameters of induration. A mean diameter of 2 mm or more is considered positive with this system. Aside from the number of positive reactions, a score is calculated which is the sum of the mean diameters of all positive reactions. Anergy is defined by the absence of any positive reaction (score 0). Patients with a score of 5 or less are considered hypoergic.

C 1740 was administered orally at a single daily dose of 8 mg (4 tablets of 2 mg) given in the morning for 5 days in 1 patient, 7 days in 10 and 15 days in 10.

Table 10.I.

Delayed cutaneous hypersensitivity to recall antigens after a short course of treatment with C 1740 in 10 anergic (no positive reactions, score 0) cancer patients

	Sex	Age	Diagnosis	Status	Number positive reactions	Score
1	F	25	Hodgkin IV Bb	Untreated	0	0
2	M	19	Hodgkin III Bb	Untreated	2	4.5
3	F	46	Ovarian tumor	Metastases	5	15.5
4	F	36	Hodgkin	Remission	3	6
5	F	54	Breast cancer	Metastases	1	2.5
6	F	26	Hodgkin	Remission	2	5
7	F	59	Metastatic cancer unknown origin	Untreated	0	0
8	M	16	Hodgkin IV Bb	Untreated	3	8
9	F	51	Non-Hodgkin lymphoma	Untreated	4	12.5
10	M	23	Hodgkin II Ab	Untreated	3	12

Table 10.II.

Delayed cutaneous hypersensitivity before and after a short course of treatment with C 1740 in 7 hypoergic (score of 5 or less) cancer patients

	Sex	Age	Diagnosis	Status	Before		After	
					Number positive reactions	Score	Number positive reactions	Score
1	M	25	Hodgkin III Bb	Untreated	1	2	3	6.5
2	F	28	Hodgkin IV Bb	Untreated	1	2	1	2
3	F	71	Non-Hodgkin lymphoma IV	Relapse	1	2	5	12
4	F	58	Breast	Untreated	2	5	4	10.5
5	F	60	Non-Hodgkin lymphoma	Relapse	2	4.5	5	16.5
6	F	47	Non Hodgkin lymphoma	Untreated	1	3	5	15.5
7	M	30	Hodgkin III Aa	Untreated	2	5	5	16.5

Before administration of C 1740, ten patients were anergic to all seven antigens (score 0), seven were hypoergic (score equal to or less than 5) and four had apparently normal DCH (score above 5). Restoration, either partial or complete, was observed in 14 out of 17 anergic and hypoergic patients (Tables 10.I. and 10.II.) with a mean score after C 1740 of 8.6 ± 5.6 compared to a pre-treatment score of 1.4 ± 1.9 ($P = 0.006$, binomial test). Three patients only showed a partial recovery of DCH switching from the anergic to an hypoergic state. Two patients with stage IV Bb Hodgkin's disease and one with liver and bone marrow metastases of unknown origin failed to respond to C 1740. Table 10.III shows the results obtained in the four patients with normal DCH. A clear enhancement of DCH was seen in 3 of 4 as shown by both the number of positive reactions and the calculated score. The only failure in this small group of patients was a 43-year-old female with metastatic breast cancer who developed clinical evidence for brain metastases during the trial (patient 3).

Table 10.III.

Delayed cutaneous hypersensitivity to recall antigens after a short course of treatment with C 1740 in 4 cancer patients with normal skin tests before treatment

	Sex	Age	Diagnosis	Status	Before		After	
					Number positive reactions	Score	Number positive reactions	Score
1	M	68	Rectum with metastases	Untreated	3	6.5	5	12.5
2	M	16	Hodgkin	Remission	2	6	6	24.5
3	F	43	Breast with metastases	Untreated	3	6	1	2
4	F	67	Breast	Metastases 3 weeks after surgery	3	9.5	5	18.5

Thus, in this open trial, DCH to recall antigens was clearly restored or enhanced in 17 of 21 patients (80%) after a short course of C 1740 given orally. The number of patients responding was similar in those who received the drug for 7 days or 15 days (8 of 10); the only patient who received C 1740 for 5 days gained four positive reactions and increased her DCH score from 2 to 12 (patient 3 in Table 10.II.). It is noteworthy that the seven patients with untreated Hodgkin's disease, a well established model of defective cell-mediated immunity, fell into the anergic and hypoergic groups, and that five of them responded to immunorestorative treatment, including four with advanced disease. No side effects were noted in our patients during the trial.

This simple clinical study clearly shows that C 1740 given per os for a short period of time has the capacity to both restore and enhance DCH to recall antigens in cancer patients. It also demonstrates that the mechanism(s) of skin anergy in tumour-bearing hosts including patients with Hodgkin's disease, may be overcome by a short course of immunotherapy. The key point in this type of study is to use a reliable and reproducible system for skin testing and the Multi-Test system fulfils these prerequisites. Attempts to modify DCH in cancer patients by short-term immunotherapy using an oral drug have been rather limited. Early studies with Levamisole reported a 25 – 70% rate of improvement of the cutaneous response to DNCB or recall antigens [1, 2, 8, 9]. However, a recently published randomized trial in a cancer population unresponsive to DNCB to determine whether Levamisole (150 mg daily $\times$ 3) given during DNCB challenge increases the conversion rate from DNCB-negative to DNCB-positive failed to show any significant influence of the drug [3]. On the other hand, the EORTC Cancer Immunology and Immunotherapy group [7] has recently reported a positive trial in patients with advanced and metastatic solid tumours with Bestatin (40 mg three times a week for 2 weeks) using the Multi-Test device. It is thus clear that immunorestoration may be obtained in a few days in a majority of cancer patients, whether this will represent a prognostic factor remains to be determined.

SUMMARY

C 1740 is a glycoproteinic extract from *Klebsiella pneumoniae*. It enhances and stimulates several parameters of the immune response in experimental animals and in humans. The compound is effective in animals even when given orally, and this route of administration proved to be devoid of any detectable toxicity. It was therefore decided to evaluate its effectiveness in vivo in man by a Phase I short-term clinical trial. We tested the capacity of C 1740 given per os for a short period of time to restore and enhance delayed cutaneous hypersensitivity to recall antigens in untreated cancer patients. 21 patients were evaluated, 13, including 7 with Hodgkin's disease, were untreated patients tested at the time of diagnosis, 5 were patients relapsing with metastases at a distance from prior treatment, and the last 3 had Hodgkin's disease in unmaintained complete remission. All these patients were unlikely to restore or enhance their skin reactivity spontaneously during the trial. No other drug was given. DCH was tested just before and after C 1740 treatment using a standardized and reproducible device of recall antigens (Multi-Test, Institut Mérieux, Lyon, France). Skin reactions were evaluated after 48 h by measuring two crossed diameters of induration. C 1740 was administered orally at a single daily dose of 8 mg for 5 days in 1 patient, 7 days in 10 and 15 days in the last 10. Restoration of DCH was observed in 14 of 17 anergic or hypoergic patients with a mean score of 8.6 ± 5.6 after C 1740 compared to a pre-treatment score of 1.4 ± 1.9 ($P = 0.006$). A clear enhancement of DCH was also seen in 3 of 4 patients with apparently normal DCH. Thus 80% of the patients positively responded to the drug and no difference was seen in the 7 day trial compared to the 15 day trial. 5 of 7 patients with Hodgkin's disease were restored. It is concluded that the drug is efficient per os and that it is capable of overcoming within a few days the mechanism(s) of skin anergy and hypoergy in cancer patients including those with Hodgkin's disease.

NOTE ADDED IN PROOF

Since this article was completed the data have been further confirmed by a controlled trial (submitted for publication).

REFERENCES

1 Brugmans, J., Schermans, V., De Cock, W., Thienpont, D., Janssen, P., Verhaegen, H., Van Nimmen, L., Louwagie, A.C. and Stevens, E. Restoration of host defence mechanisms in man by levamisole. Life Sci. 13, 1499, 1973.
2 Hirshaut, Y., Pinsky, C., Marquardt, H. and Oettgen, H.F. Effects of levamisole on delayed hypersensitivity reactions in cancer patients. Proc. Am. Assoc. Cancer Res. 14, 109, 1973.
3 Hirshaut, Y., Pinsky, C.M., Frydecka, I., Wanebo, H.M., Passe, S., Mike, V. and Oettgen, H.F. Effect of short-term levamisole therapy on delayed hypersensitivity. Cancer 45, 362, 1980.
4 Kniker, W.T., Anderson, C.T. and Roumiantzeff M. The Multi-Test system: a standardized approach to evaluation of delayed hypersensitivity and cell-mediated immunity. Ann. Allergy 43, 73, 1979.
5 Lesourd, B.M., Roumiantzeff, M., Moulias, R., Biron, G. and Kniker, W.T. Reproducibility of delayed cutaneous hypersensitivity (DCH) measured by Multi-Test. XIth Congress of the European Academy of Allergology and Clinical Immunology Vienna, Austria, 1980.
6 Leventhal, B.G. Quantitation of delayed hypersensitivity responses in the skin: a new device. Meeting on Immunological Aspects of Experimental and Clinical Cancer, Tel Aviv, Israel, 1979.
7 Serrou, B., Cupissol, D., Flad, H., Goutner, A., Lang, J.M., Spirzglas, H., Plagne, R., Beltzer, M., Chollet, P. and Mathe, G. Phase I evaluation of Bestatin in patients bearing advanced solid tumors. Internat. J. Immunopharmacol. 2, 168, 1980.
8 Tripodi, D., Parks, L.C., Brugmans, J. Drug-induced restoration of cutaneous delayed hypersensitivity in anergic patients with cancer. N. Engl. J. Med. 289, 354, 1973.
9 Webster D.J.T. and Hughes L.E. Levamisole. Lancet i, 389, 1975.

CHAPTER 11

The current status of cyclomunine

Nicole Simon-Lavoine

Laboratoire Servier, Neuilly (France)

11.1. INTRODUCTION

The use of pharmaceutical agents to manipulate the immune system has emerged as a real possibility. Among the candidates for such purposes cyclomunine is of interest to experimental and clinical immunologists. This report summarizes the experimental work that has already been done and illustrates that cyclomunine is an immunomodulator worthy of attention.

11.2. PROPERTIES

Cyclomunine is a hexacyclodepsipeptide which was originally extracted from *Fusarium equiseti* (Commonwealth Mycological Institute stain No. 213 107). It is hardly water soluble, a fact probably related to its cyclic structure, and its molecular weight has been estimated by mass spectrography as 500.

11.3. EFFECTS

The effects of cyclomunine have been evaluated in conventional immunological assay systems, both in vitro and in vivo, at low doses and high doses, and the following sections describe the results.

11.3.1. *Macrophages*

Cyclomunine stimulates macrophage production when administered intravenously in aqueous and ethanolic solution at concentrations at less than 1 μg kg^{-1} and 1 mg kg^{-1} respectively.

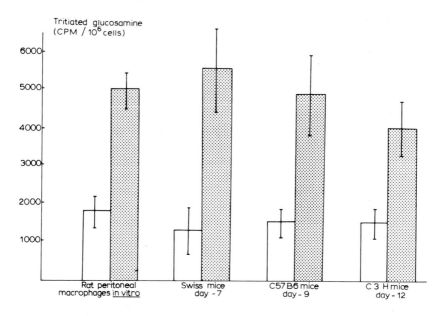

Fig. 11.1. In vitro glucosamine incorporation either by peritoneal macrophages after 6 h incubation with 100 ng tritiated glucosamine per ml (rat macrophages, left hand bars), or by peritoneal macrophages from mice treated at the indicated period with 100 ng cyclomunine solution intravenously (three pairs of right hand bars). Open bars, control macrophages; stippled bars, cyclomunine-treated macrophages or animals.

Fig. 11.1. shows the amount of radiolabelled glucosamine incorporated into cultivated macrophages in the presence of cyclomunine in vitro, or in vivo on peritoneal resident macrophages freshly explanted from mice prior to intravenous treatment with cyclomunine at different times before the assay. In all the cases, there is a significant increase in the incorporation of tritiated glucosamine.

Fig. 11.2. shows the significant chemoattractant effect of cyclomunine in an in vitro assay. Cyclomunine, at the indicated concentrations, is located in the lower part of the modified boyden chambers.

The internal bars are chambers where the chemotactic gradient is nullified by the addition of cyclomunine to both the upper and lower part of the chambers.

Macrophages from mice treated with cyclomunine display an increased bactericidal capacity against *Staphylococcus aureus* (Fig. 11.3.). About one log less replicating bacteria was eventually recovered from experimental cultures as compared to control cultures.

The effect of macrophages on a rat tumor cell line can be seen in Fig. 11.4., in vivo and in vitro, and in all cases there was a significant increase in the tumoricidal effect of macrophages after treatment with cyclomunine.

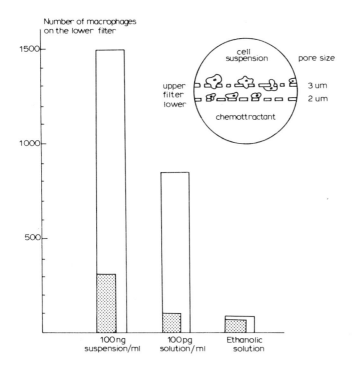

Fig. 11.2. Chemotactic activity of cyclomunine on rat purified resident macrophages, measured by the double polycarbonate filter method in Boyden chambers. Open bars, Boyden chambers with chemoattractant in lower compartment only; stippled bars, Boyden chambers with chemoattractant in upper and lower compartments.

11.3.2. *Lymphocytes*

The effects of cyclomunine on lymphocytes have been tested in vitro in two systems: blastic transformation induced by mitogens, antigens and allogenic stimulation; and the suppressive effect of Con A pre-stimulated lymphocytes on a mixed lymphocyte culture, a system which is a measure of the activity of T suppressor lymphocytes.

Fig. 11.5. shows the effects of cyclomunine ($2.5 - 10$ µg ml^{-1}) on murine lymphocytes stimulated with allogenic cells, PHA or Con A. A significant effect was observed at concentrations of cyclomunine from 4 to 6 µg ml^{-1}. The same results were obtained on human lymphocytes. Fig. 11.6. shows a similar inhibition of PPD (purified protein derivative) sensitive human lymphocytes at 5, 10 and 20 µg ml^{-1}.

The viability of T, B and non T-non B lymphoblastoid cell lines, incubated with various concentrations of cyclomunine is shown on Fig. 11.7. Cyclomunine was toxic at 1 µg ml^{-1} to 90% of Raji cells; 5 µg ml^{-1} killed 80% of the T cell line and 90% of the non T-non B cell line. Thus cyclomunine at low doses, in vitro, has a major antilymphoblastic activity. This cytotoxicity is highly specific, as 10 µg ml^{-1}

144

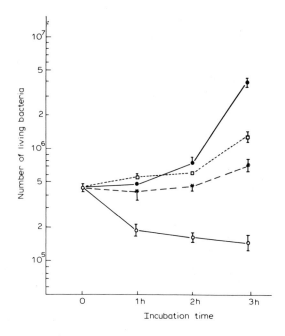

Fig. 11.3. In vitro bactericidal activity of rat peritoneal macrophages against *Staphylococcus aureus* 8 days after intravenous injection of cyclomunine. Filled circle, control growth; open square, control macrophages; star, cyclomunine (250 μg); open circles, cyclomunine (100 ng).

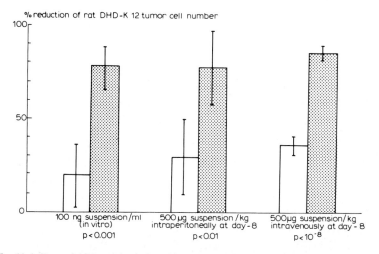

Fig. 11.4. Tumoricidal activity induced in normal rat peritoneal macrophages by cyclomunine, against the rat adenocarcinoma DHD-K12 cell line (a gift from M-S. and F. Martin, Dijon). The percentage of tumoral cell reduction is calculated against macrophage-free cultures of tumoral cells in the same medium. The open bars represent control macrophages; the stippled areas cyclomunine-stimulated macrophages or animals.

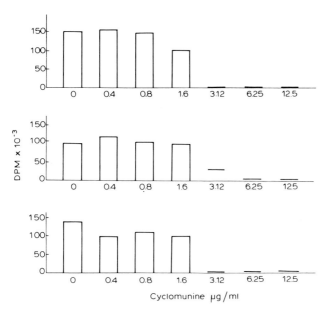

Fig. 11.5. Effect of cyclomunine on murine lymphocyte proliferation induced by allogenic cells (top); PHA (centre); and Con A (bottom).

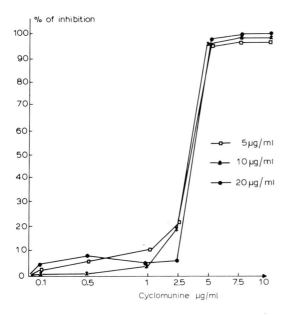

Fig. 11.6. Inhibition of thymidine incorporation in PPD-stimulated human lymphocyte cultures in the presence of cyclomunine. Open squares, 5 µg ml^{-1}; stars, 10 µg ml^{-1}; filled circles, 20 µg ml^{-1}.

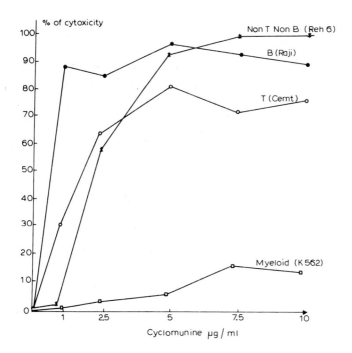

Fig. 11.7. Cytotoxicity of lymphoblastoid cell lines.

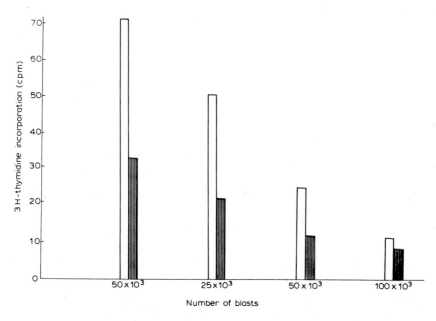

Fig. 11.8. Suppression of Con A-pre-stimulated lymphoblasts. Open bars, Con A alone; lined bars, Con A + cyclomunine (1 μg ml⁻¹).

will kill only 10% of a myeloid cell line and less than 50% of stimulated lymphocytes.

Lymphocytes incubated with optimal amounts of Con A for 48 h then washed, will exert a measurable inhibitory activity on an on-going allogenic lymphocyte stimulation. This T cell suppressive activity was also sensitive to cyclomunine.

Con A pre-stimulated lymphocytes incubated with 1 ng of cyclomunine and then washed were more suppressive than untreated Con A pre-stimulated lymphocytes (Fig. 11.8.).

Increasing numbers of Con A pre-stimulated lymphoblasts were added to the mixed lymphocytes cultures. On average, thymidine uptake was 50% less in cultures to which cyclomunine-pretreated cells were added.

Nuclear refringence testing permits the detection of early alterations of the stimulated lymphocyte nuclei. A decrease in the refringence is observed in stimulated cells, due to a dispersion of the chromatine. Using this test, low doses of cyclomunine ranging from 1 pg to 1 ng mg^{-1} significantly decreased the refringence, but high doses, ranging from 1 to 10 µg ml^{-1} increased such nuclear refringence (Fig. 11.9.).

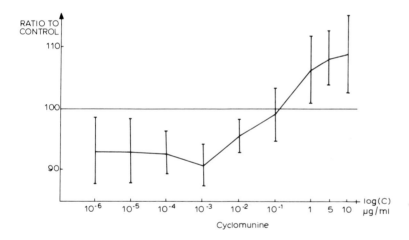

Fig. 11.9. Early modification of nuclear refringence after short incubation with cyclomunine.

11.3.3. *Thymus*

Cyclomunine as early as four days after a single intraperitoneal injection (12.5 mg kg^{-1}) has a striking impact on the thymus as indicated by: a definite increase in the medullary to cortical ratio; a significant increase in the number of Hassal's bodies; and an alteration in the aspect of such Hassal's bodies where cells appear distinctly turgid but are not destroyed.

Fig. 11.10. represents these effects. It can be seen that the progressive increase in the number of modified Hassal's bodies reaches a 2–5 fold peak between days 14 and 21.

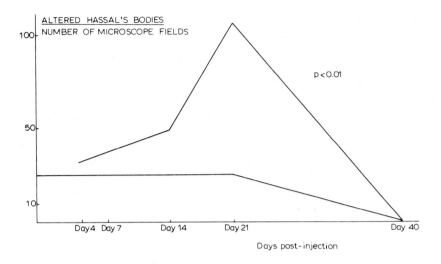

Fig. 11.10. Effect of a single intraperitoneal injection of 12.5 mg kg^{-1} on the thymus of 6-week-old Swiss mice. The number of altered Hassal's bodies were counted in microscope fields. Upper line, cyclomunine-treated mice; lower line, control.

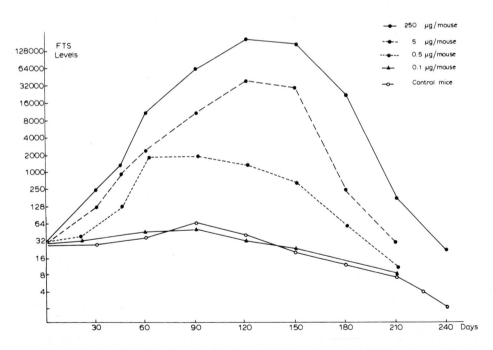

Fig. 11.11. Effect of a single injection of various doses of cyclomunine on the FTS levels in normal young mice.

Another effect is that rather large vacuoles appear within thymic epithelial cells which stain positively with PAS. These abnormal vacuoles are clearly visible under the electron microscope. In contrast with the Hassal's bodies alterations, these altered epithelial vacuoles persist beyond day forty.

Because of these modifications, we then looked for alterations of thymic secretion products in the serum of treated mice and found that in normal mice the FTS (Facteur Thymique Sérique; thymic humoral factor) level declines after 6 months but in NZB mice the level decreases as soon as three weeks after birth.

After treatment, a most striking and sustained rise in FTS levels is seen in animals following a single injection with a peak between days 90 and 160, reaching titers as high as a thousand fold increase over the basal levels and even more (Fig. 11.11.). This effect is dose dependent. No effect was seen with 0.1 μg ml^{-1}.

This major rise in FTS levels is also seen in NZB mice. Immunofluorescent studies with an anti-FTS fluorescinated antibody showed up to 3-fold increase in the number of FTS-secreting epithelial cells. (Fig. 11.12.). Thus, cyclomunine induced major alteration in the thymus.

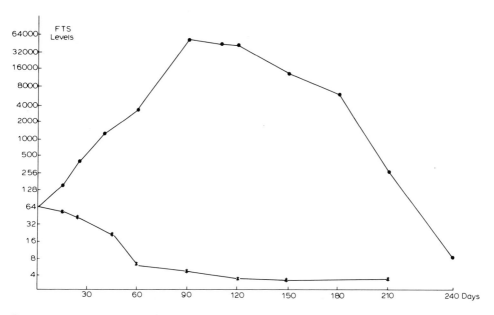

Fig. 11.12. Evolution of FTS levels after a single injection of cyclomunine (250 μg per mouse) in 3-week-old NZB mice. Upper line, experimental; lower line, control.

11.3.4. *Immune function*

A number of immune functions in animals treated with cyclomunine were evaluated, as follows:

1. IgM antibody response to sheep red blood cell after a primary in vivo

150

immunization.

2. Capacity of mice to survive a flu or an encephalomyocarditis infection.
3. Kidney or skin allograft acceptance.
4. Weight of the spleens of irradiated mice injected with spleen cells from A H$_2$ non compatible strain.

As can be seen from Fig. 11.13, there is a significant increase in the number of plaque-forming cells (PFC) from the spleen of mice receiving low doses of cyclomunine prior to or simultaneously with an immunizing dose of sheep red blood cells (SRBC).

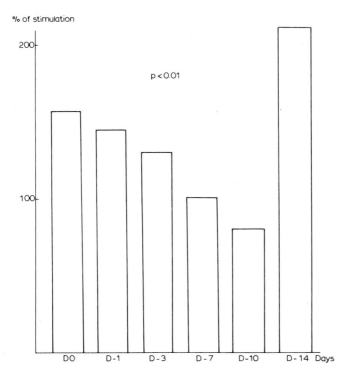

Fig. 11.13. Response of the spleen of mice receiving 0.0025 μg kg^{-1} cyclomunine prior to or simultaneously with an immunizing dose of sheep red blood cells.

However, Fig. 11.13. shows a decrease in PFC in animals receiving higher doses of cyclomunine, with a 50% reduction when cyclomunine was given 7 days before immunization (Fig. 11.14.).

With such high doses one could significantly suppress a graft versus host reaction in mice (Table 11.I.) Animals were treated with 12.5 μg kg^{-1} (equal to 250 μg per mouse) from day minus to day plus seven; they were then irradiated and received spleen cells from a non-compatible mouse strain. At day seven after engrafting, the ratio of the spleen weight to the whole mouse weight was calculated. The difference between untreated and treated mice at high doses reaches statistical significance, establishing that cyclomunine is active in this most potent allogenic stimulation of a graft versus host reaction.

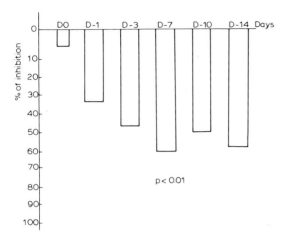

Fig. 11.14. Anti-SRBC-IgM response to 12.5 µg kg⁻¹ cyclomunine.

Table 11.I.

Graft versus host reaction after daily treatment with cyclomunine

Daily dose of cyclomunine per mouse	Spleen/body weight ratio	No. mice in each group
0	2.24 ± 0.49 *	17
2.5 µg	2.15 ± 0.49	17
250 µg	1.75 ± 0.41 *	14

*Results are means ± SE. * $P < 0.01$ (Student's t test).

The anti-allogenic effect of high doses of cyclomunine was more impressive in organ allografts since skin allograft survival in mice was significantly prolonged and survival of Wistar kidney allografts in Lewis rats treated with 12.5 mg/kg per day intraperitoneally was significantly prolonged (Fig. 11.15.).

Thus to conclude, at high doses, cyclomunine exhibits a definite anti-rejection effect in the various allogenic systems.

Cyclomunine was tested for its antiviral activity in whole animals. Cyclomunine at low doses can influence the outcome of two viral infections experimentally inoculated into mice. As a preventive measure, pretreatment of animals with aerosols of cyclomunine for 8 days before challenge with Hong-Kong influenza

152

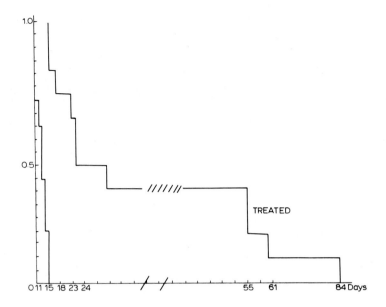

Fig. 11.15. Survival of Wistar kidney allografts in Lewis rats treated with cyclomunine 12.5 mg per kg per day, intraperitoneally.

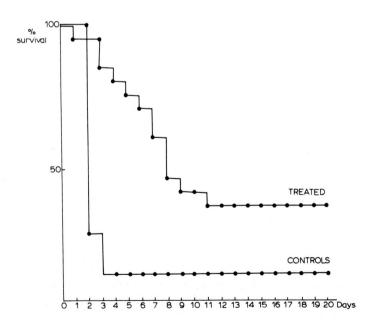

Fig. 11.16. Protection of mice against influenza by pretreatment with aerosols of cyclomunine.

virus significantly protected the pretreated animals (Fig. 11.16). The animals inhaled an equivalent total dose of 1 μg. The early mortality rate was most significantly altered in treated mice. Of great interest was the finding that cyclomunine at low doses in a single injection had marked effect in interferon-mediated protection against the encephalomyocarditis virus (Fig. 11.17.).

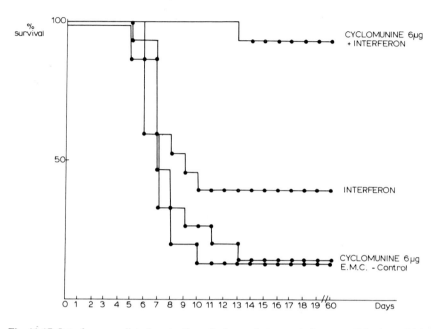

Fig. 11.17. Interferon-mediated protection of mice against encephalomyocarditis virus with low doses o cyclomunine.

Mice received 6 μg of cyclomunine i.v. 24 h before an exposure to 151 LD 50 EMC virus given i.p. Interferon was administered 1 h after inoculation. The potentiation by cyclomunine of the moderate protective effect of interferon given alone is quite obvious. Similar experiments were repeated and gave identical results in three different series of such experiments.

Taken together the available data indicate that cyclomunine is acting as an immunomodulator, as it seems to show different effects on the immune system according to the dosage used.

11.4. CONCLUSIONS

The doses of 5–10 μg ml^{-1} in vitro and 12.5 mg kg^{-1} in vivo cyclomunine suppress mitogen and antigen-induced blastic transformation of lymphocytes, prolong kidney and skin allografts, reduce graft-versus-host-reactions and decrease the PFC response to SRBC.

At low doses (10^{-6}–10^{-3} μg ml^{-1} in vitro; 1.25–500 μg kg^{-1} in vivo) cyclomunine stimulates metabolic and biological activities of macrophages, increases the primary response to SRBC, enhances T suppressor function in a Con A and MLC assays and potentiates interferon-mediated protection against EMC virus.

ACKNOWLEDGEMENTS

I should like to acknowledge the participation of the following workers: J.F. Bach, M. Dardenne, D. Riveau, P. Niaudet, G. Beaurain; P. Burtin, G. Lespinats; A. Capron, M. Joseph; C. Chany, I. Cerruti; A. Desplaces, J. Dufer; R. Fontanges; J.W. Hadden, R. Faanes, W. Kreis, J. Raaf; J.M. Lang; F. Oberling; J. Leibovitch; G. Mathe, I. Florentin; A. Pompidou; G. Renoux; B. Serrou; J.L. Touraine, J. Amiel, J.M. Dubernard, J. Navarro.

CHAPTER 12

Modulation of the immune response by cimetidine

B. Serrou[a], A. Rey[a], D. Cupissol[a],
C. Thierry[a], C. Estève[a] and C. Rosenfeld[b]

[a]Laboratoire d'Immunopharmacologie des Tumeurs INSERM U 236, ERA-CNRS
No. 844, Centre Paul Lamarque, Montpellier and Département de Cultures et
Production de Cellules Humaines, INSERM U 50, ICIG, Hôpital Paul Brousse,
14-16, Av. P. Vaillant Couturier, Villejuif (France)

12.1. INTRODUCTION

Cimetidine is a drug widely employed in the treatment of gastritis and ulcers [13]. It
acts on the H_2 surface receptors of a large number of cells [18]. Several recent
studies suggest that these receptors are found on lymphocytes [23,25] and that such
lymphocytes are part of a suppressor subpopulation presenting Fc receptor for IgG
[14, 28]. Moreover, some studies indicate that cimetidine may increase PFC
antibody production when injected before or with antigen in either normal or
tumor-bearing animals [11]. This results in prolonged survival time for these
tumor-bearing animals. Cimetidine has been suggested to retard allograft rejection,
but these results are quite contradictory [8,9,10,19,24], and to favor the growth of
gastric tumor [15,20]. Taken as a whole, the results suggest an immunomodulating
role for this drug [29].

The information accrued as a result of these studies would appear to justify
further investigation of cimetidine effects on certain immune functions of human
lymphocytes in vitro.

12.2. MATERIAL AND METHODS

12.2.1. Isolation of lymphocytes

Peripheral blood lymphocytes were separated from whole blood by the method of
Boyum [3] using a Ficoll-metrizoate gradient of specific gravity 1.077.

12.2.2. Auto-rosette forming cell (ARFC) assay

The technique employed was that of Caraux et. al. [6,7]. Briefly, 0.20 ml of lymphocyte suspension (10^7 cells ml^{-1}) was preincubated for 30 min at 4°C with 0.05 ml of autologous serum.

Autologous erythrocytes (auto-RBC) (3×10^8 ml^{-1}) were added to the lymphocyte serum suspension which was centrifuged at $200 \times g$ for 5 min and incubated overnight at +4°C. ARFC were counted the following day using a hemocytometer. An auto-rosette was defined as a lymphocyte binding three or more auto RBCs.

12.2.3. NK activity

This parameter was evaluated using cells from the K562 [16] line originating from chronic myeloid leukemia. The cells were tagged with ^{51}Cr by incubation at 37°C for 2 h. The cells were then washed and constituted the target cell for the NK assay. 10×10^3 target cells were incubated at 37°C for 18 h in contact with test lymphocytes. The effector/target (E/T) cell ratios employed were 6/1, 12/1, 25/1 and 50/1.

Results are expressed as % cytotoxicity calculated as follows:

$$NK(\%) = \frac{R - RS}{RM - RS} \times 100$$

R is the radioactivity in the supernatant at the end of incubation; RS is the radioactivity of supernatant in a test to which no lymphocytes were added (spontaneous cpm release); RM is the radioactivity observed following complete lysis by hydrochloric acid (total cpm).

12.2.4. Mitogen responsiveness

We used a method previously described [27]. Briefly, 100 µl of the lymphocyte suspension adjusted to 1×10^6 ml^{-1} was incubated with 50 µl of the appropriate mitogen (PHA, Con A or PWM) at 37°C in a humid atmosphere for 72 h. 16 h before termination of the culture, 50 µl of tritiated thymidine containing 0.2 µCi were added to the culture. The cultures were then filtered, dried and their radioactivity measured.

12.2.5. Mixed lymphocyte culture

The technique has been previously described [26]. Briefly the stimulating cells were blocked with mitomycine C (Sigma). A ratio of 1/1 (i.e. 5×10^5 stimulating cells/5 $\times 10^5$ cells stimulated) was used. Culture time was 5 days. Radioactivity of [^{3}H]thymidine incorporated in the previous 16 h was then measured in the cultures.

12.2.6. Effects of cimetidine (SKF Lab.)

Cimetidine was incubated for 1 h at 37°C with lymphocyte suspension before each test at 10^{-3}M, 10^{-4}M, 10^{-6}M per ml per 10^7 lymphocytes.

12.3. RESULTS

12.3.1. The effect of cimetidine on ARFC

The results (Table 12.I.) show that cimetidine did not alter ARFC levels in healthy subjects. In contrast, it significantly increased ARFC numbers in tumor patients with subnormal levels. This effect was more significantly demonstrated for patients with

Table 12.I.

Effect of cimetidine on auto-rosette forming cells

		ARFC (%)
Control (C)		27 ± 3.01
Cancer patients		
High level	(HL)	19 ± 2.84
Low level	(LL)	9 ± 1.41
Cimetidine		
10^{-3} M	C	29 ± 3.53
	HL	24 ± 2.74
	LL	16 ± 2.21
10^{-4} M	C	27 ± 2.91
	HL	22 ± 2.37
	LL	14 ± 2.03
10^{-6}M	C	25 ± 2.44
	HL	20 ± 2.39
	LL	11 ± 2.01

extremely low ARFC levels, in whom a very significant in vitro augmentation can be induced in the presence of 10^{-3}M cimetidine. No toxicity was noted for lymphocytes at this concentration.

12.3.2. The effect of cimetidine on NK activity

We have observed a relatively weak, but significant rise in NK activity. However, this increase was less significant as compared with that noted for bestatin, isoprinosine or interferon.

Table 12 II

Effects of cimetidine on lymphocyte mitogen responsiveness

	PHA		PWM		Con A	
	dpm ± SD	%	dpm ± SD	%	dpm ± SD	%
Control	114 657 ± 2500		121 672 ± 2300		137 628 ± 2100	
Cimetidine						
10^{-3} M	191 321 ± 3900	66	198 221 ± 3500	62	216 521 ± 3100	57
10^{-4} M	178 434 ± 2400	55	176 745 ± 1950	45	194 498 ± 3100	41
10^{-6} M	153 829 ± 2700	34	151 928 ± 2200	24	166 341 ± 2600	20

12.3.3. The effect of cimetidine on lymphocyte mitogen responsiveness

There was a very significant increase for PHA. PWM and Con A response for lymphocytes from normal control subjects (Table 12.2.). This effect was directly dose dependent, the most efficacious dose therefore being 10^{-3} M. This concentration yielded increased responses of 66%, 52% and 57% respectively for PHA, PWM and Con A.

Table 12.III.

Effect of cimetidine on MLC

	MLC	
	dpm ± SD	%
Control	81 324 ± 1700	
Cimetidine		
10^{-3} M	143 956 ± 2100	77
10^{-4} M	121 278 ± 2200	49
10^{-6} M	117 669 ± 1900	44

12.3.4. The effect of cimetidine on MLC

These results (Table 12.III.) parallel those obtained for the mitogen assays with the most effective dose at 10^{-3}M. A 77% increase was observed compared to control values. Here again no cytotoxicity was encountered.

12.4. DISCUSSION

The results show that cimetidine is capable of modulating certain immune functions in vitro. To begin with, there is an increase in ARFC, especially noted for the immunodepressed cancer patient presenting low ARFC. It has been found [21] that ARFC correspond to two subpopulations, one of which forms autorosettes after 1 h (probably immature T lymphocytes), the other forming auto-rosettes following overnight incubation (thought to be lymphocytes with an Fc receptor for IgM). These cells respond the same in autologous or allogenic mixed lymphocyte cultures. These results for ARFC parallel those obtained for mixed cultures tested with cimetidine. The most significant increase in the mixed-culture response was noted for 10^{-3} M cimetidine. Again, there was no detectable cytotoxicity. These results are particularly interesting since MLC represents a well-characterized immune function. This T cell effect is corroborated by mitogen response, which also demonstrates a parallel increase. Once again, the maximum effect was observed for the 10^{-3} M concentration.

The present results agree with those of different authors who suggest that cimetidine modulates the immune response [12], particularly the PFC response to antigens such as sheep red blood cells [11]. This was observed for both normal and tumor-bearing animals and was associated with prolonged survival of tumor animals [11].

Taken together, these results suggest a possible modulatory role for cimetidine in the immune response. These findings agree with previous results suggesting prolonged survival of allografts [8,9,19,24] and a permissive role concerning gastric tumors [15,20]. In fact, there appears to be a great number of substances which act as modulators on the immune system and whose action depends on the context into which the agent enters. This would include the relationship between time of injection and the antigenic environment which exists, the dose employed, and the immune status of the organism at time of injection. The interaction of all these factors can lead to completely opposite effects for the same drug. The fact that cimetidine acts on ARFC and mixed cultures suggests that its target is the T lymphocyte. We have shown that increased ARFC levels are usually accompanied by decreased suppressor activity in the immunodepressed, advanced solid tumor patient [7].

The target cell for cimetidine could be concerned with the T helper lymphocyte, or mostly the T suppressor lymphocyte bearing H_2 receptors [14], but, as some authors have noted, may also involve the B lymphocyte and macrophage [23]. More in depth studies have shown that this drug possesses minimal toxicity [4] and exerts an effect on other cell types such as circulating leukocytes and may therefore have repercussions on inflammatory responses and the productions of different substances such as prostaglandins [4]. Whatever the final analysis, at present the wide clinical use of cimetidine, the paradoxical results concerning the modulation of the immune response [1,2,5,10] and the discovery that circulating lymphocytes possess H_2 receptors, demand a more precise evaluation of cimetidine's immuno-modulatory effects. It is very possible that this drug could eventually become an element within the therapeutic arsenal of agents modulating human immune response, not only in cancer, but other types of pathologies as well.

REFERENCES

1. Askenase, P.W. Histamine – 2 antagonist inhibition of delayed hypersensitivity (DH). Clin. Res., 25, 481, 1977.
2. Avella, J., Madsew, J.E., Binder, H.J. and Askenase, P.W. Effect of histamine H_2-receptor antagonists on delayed hypersensitivity. Lancet, i, 624, 1978.
3. Boyum, A. Separation of leukocytes from blood and bone marrow. Scand. J. Clin. Lab. Invest., 21, 97, 1968.
4. Burland, W.L., Duncan, W.A.M., Hesselbo, T., Mills, J.G., Sharpe, P.C., Haggie, S.J. and Wyllie, J.H. Pharmacological evaluation of cimetidine, a new H_2 receptor antagonist in healthy man. Br. J. Clin. Pharmacol. 2, 481, 1975.
5. Calvo, D.B., Mavligit, G.M., Hersh, E.M. and Patt, Y.Z. Immuno-restoration and/or immuno augmentation of local xenogeneic graft versus host reaction with cimetidine. Proc. AACR, 21, 841 (abstract), 1980.
6. Caraux, J., Thierry, C., Esteve, C., Flores, G., Lodise, R. and Serrou, B. Human autologous rosettes. I. Mechanism of binding of autologous erythrocytes by T cells. Cell. Immunol. 45, 36, 1979.
7. Caraux, J., Thierry, C. and Serrou, B. Human autologous rosettes. II. Prognostic significance of variations in autologous rosette forming cells in the peripheral blood of cancer patients. J. Natl. Cancer Inst. 63, 593, 1979.
8. Charpentier, B. and Fries, D. Cimetidine and renal-allograft rejection. Lancet, i, 1265, 1978.
9. Doherty, C.C. and McGeown, M.G. Cimetidine and renal–allograft rejection. Lancet, i, 705, 1978.
10. Festen, H.P.M., Berden, J.H.M. and Koewe, R.A.P. Cimetidine does not accelerate skin graft rejection in mice. Clin. Exp. Immunol., 40, 193, 1980.
11. Friedman, H. Immunomodulating effects of cimetidine. in Augmenting Agents in Cancer Therapy (Hersh, E.M., Chirigos, M.A. and Mastrangelo, M.J. Eds) Vol. 16, p. 417, 1981. Raven Press; New York.
12. Gifford, R.R.M., Hatfield, S.M. and Schmidtke, J.R. Cimetidine induced modulation of human lymphocyte blastogenesis. Proc. AACR, 21, 661 (abstract), 1980.
13. Gray, G.R., McKenzie, I., Smith, I.S., Crean, G.P. and Gillespie, G. Oral cimetidine in severe duodenal ulceration. Lancet, i, 4, 1977.
14. Gupta, S., Fernandes, G., Rocklin, R. and Good, R. Histamine receptors on Human T cell subsets. in New Trends in Human Immunology and Cancer Immunotherapy (Serrou, B., and Rosenfeld C. Eds), pp. 36-47, 1980. Doin, Paris.
15. Hawker, P.C., Muscroftt, J. and Keighley, M.R.B. Gastric cancer after cimetidine in patient with two negative pretreatment biopsies. Lancet, i, 709, 1980.
16. Lozzio, C.B. and Lozzio, B.B. Cytotoxicity of a factor isolated from human spleen. J. Natl. Cancer Inst., 50, 535, 1973.
17. Plaut, M., Lichtenstein, L.M., Gillespie, E. and Henney, C.S. Studies on the mechanism of lymphocytes mediated cytolysis. IV. Specificity of the histamine receptor on effector T cells. J. Immunol. 111, 389, 1973.
18. Plaut, M., Lichtenstein, L.M. and Henney, C.S. Properties of a subpopulation of T cells bearing histamine receptors. J. Clin. Invest. 55, 856, 1975.
19. Primack, W.A. Cimetidine and renal-allograft rejection. Lancet, i, 676, 1978.
20. Reed, P.I., Cassel, P.G. and Walters, C.L. Gastric cancer in patients who have taken cimetidine. Lancet, i, 1234, 1979.
21. Rey, A., Rucheton, M., Caraux, J., Esteve, C., Thierry, C. and Serrou, B. Auto-rosette forming cells : Functional evaluation. 1981, in press.
22. Randolph, W.C., Osborne, V.L., Walkewstein, S.S. and Intoccia, A.P. High pressure liquid

chromatographic analysis of cimetidine, a histamine H_2-receptor antagonist in blood and mice. J. Pharm, Sci., 66, 1148, 1977.

23 Rocklin, R.E. Modulation of cellular immune response in vivo and in vitro by histamine receptor bearing lymphocytes. J. Clin. Invest., 57, 1051, 1976.

24 Rudge, C.J., Jones, R.H., Bewick, M., Weston, M.J. and Parsons, V. Cimetidine and renal-allograft rejection. Lancet, i, 775, 1978.

25 Saxon, A., Morledge, V.D. and Bonavida, B. Histamine receptor leucocytes (HRL). Organ and lymphoid subpopulation distribution in man. Clin. Exp. Immunol. 28, 394, 1977.

26 Serrou, B., Thierry, C., Turc., J.M., and Valles, H. Markers and immunological responsiveness of fresh and frozen-thawed human lymphocytes. in Cryoimmunology (Simatos, D., Strong, D.M. and Turc, J.M. Eds), Colloques et Séminaires: INSERM 62, 93, 1976.

27 Thierry, C. and Serrou, B. La stimulation blastique des lymphocytes par les mitogènes. in Microtechnique de Stimulation Blastique des Lymphocytes chez l'Homme. (Serrou, B. Ed), Colloques et Séminaires, INSERM 35, 35, 1974.

28 Verhaegen, H., De Cok, W., and Decree, J. Histamine receptor bearing peripheral T lymphocytes in patients with allergies. J. Allergy Clin. Immunol., 59, 266, 1977.

29 Wang, S.R. and Zweiman, B. Histamine suppression of human lymphocyte responses to mitogens Cell. Immunol., 36, 28, 1978.

Subject index